SLOW
SEX

"Like everything else in this fast-forward world, our sex lives have been infected by the virus of hurry. *Slow Sex* is the perfect antidote. With warmth and wisdom, Diana Richardson shows how slowing down in the bedroom can bring us better sex, better relationships, and a better world. What are you waiting for? The time has come to unleash your inner tortoise in the bedroom!"

CARL HONORÉ, AUTHOR OF *IN PRAISE OF SLOWNESS*

"How rare it is for a book to appear about sex and sensuality with a truly fresh and innovative approach. Diana Richardson has crafted a masterpiece that is warm, evocative, timely, and accessible to everyone. Her wise and inviting style will welcome you into a fascinating new world where your experience of sexuality will be forever changed. If you've wanted just one book that could give you the most simple and powerful access into the ancient, beautiful world of Tantra, here it is . . ."

MARC DAVID, AUTHOR OF *THE SLOW DOWN DIET* AND FOUNDER OF THE INSTITUTE FOR THE PSYCHOLOGY OF EATING

SLOW SEX

The Path to Fulfilling and Sustainable Sexuality

DIANA RICHARDSON

Destiny Books

Rochester, Vermont • Toronto, Canada

Destiny Books
One Park Street
Rochester, Vermont 05767
www.DestinyBooks.com

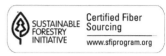

Text paper is SFI certified

Destiny Books is a division of Inner Traditions International

Library of Congress Cataloging-in-Publication Data

Richardson, Diana.
 Slow sex : the path to fulfilling and sustainable sexuality / Diana Richardson.
  p. cm.
 ISBN 978-1-59477-367-9 (pbk.)
 1. Sexual intercourse. 2. Sex instruction. I. Title.
 HQ31.R48 2011
 613.9'6—dc22

                                                                2010042853

Printed and bound in the United States by Lake Book Manufacturing
The text paper is SFI certified. The Sustainable Forestry Initiative® program
promotes sustainable forest management.

10   9   8   7   6   5   4   3   2

Text design and layout by Virginia Scott Bowman
This book was typeset in Garamond Premier Pro with Perpetua, Avant Garde, and
    Swiss used as display typefaces
Artwork in chapters 4 and 5 prepared by Alfredo Hernando, Madrid, Spain.
Artwork in chapter 10 (with the exception of fig. 10.3) prepared by Gabriel
    Tempesta, Wolcott, Vermont, **www.tempestart.homestead.com**

To send correspondence to the author of this book, mail a first-class letter to the
author c/o Inner Traditions • Bear & Company, One Park Street, Rochester, VT
05767, and we will forward the communication or contact the author directly at
www.livinglove.com or **info@livinglove.com**.

To the Revolution that Heralds Our Evolution

Recently, I invited my longest-standing erotic partner to read Diana's book on conscious sex. Our "love connection" had been dead for more than twenty years. No ecstatic experience left, dead, dead, dead.

We naturally, effortlessly started following the instructions in the book, inspired and transported by something in it, something new and loving, some energy and wisdom emanating from its pages. Lo and behold, we spent the next two weeks in five- to nine-hour sessions, reaching a state so beautiful I wanted to stay there forever.

I had never understood why people called sex "making love" and here we were making, within ourselves and between us, a tangible love energy. My intelligent penis "knew" when my partner's vagina was open. It knew to stay cool, in that receptive state where *it* was guiding me, *it* knew when to penetrate and how. My heart was in joy, my whole body felt touched by her vagina. We remained for hours in this glow, losing all sense of time. A few times I felt her heart touching my penis from very deep in the vagina. She had not self-lubricated in decades; she had lost contact with the vagina, now *it* became alive. At one point she said, glowing in deep appreciation and love: "I feel like a woman for the first time in my life."

CONTENTS

ACKNOWLEDGMENTS

My heartfelt thanks to Marc David, whose book *The Slow Down Diet* arrived in my life as if by divine hand to become an inspiration far beyond anything I had ever anticipated. I am very grateful for his generosity in allowing me to use his words, which appear as short extracts throughout this book.

I also wish to extend my deepest gratitude to the couples I have met in my workshops over the years for their trust, and for giving me endless inspiration and encouragement by being living and loving endorsements that man and woman thrive and flourish on slow sex.

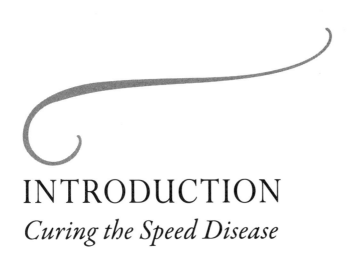

INTRODUCTION
Curing the Speed Disease

In keeping with the emerging Slow Food movement, I was delighted when my publisher suggested that I write a book entitled *Slow Sex*. This is a subject that is dear to my heart. My partner, Michael, and I have been facilitating weeklong "Making Love" retreats for couples since 1993. During these retreats we teach couples to take a fresh approach toward sex—to slow down and be fully present to each moment while having sex together, rather than practice more active sex that strives so intensely toward orgasm that it misses the subtler nuances of union along the way.

In short, we teach couples how to cultivate a slow sex practice. It is crystal clear to both of us that when couples engage in sex at a more leisurely pace, in which each moment is slowly savored and relished with awareness, they experience more sensitivity, sensuality, and satisfaction. Afterward they feel deeply nourished by love, empowered as a couple, and significantly, equally empowered as individuals too.

Recently a friend suggested I read *The Slow Down Diet: Eating for Pleasure, Energy, and Weight Loss* by Marc David. This book turned out to be an exceptional source of information, insight, and inspiration—not just in relation to food, but also in relation to sex. Marc David is a professional nutritionist with a master's degree in the psychology of eating. Through his own personal experiences in the practice of yoga, he became acquainted with the existence of eight universal metabolic enhancers that are *transubstantial,* meaning "above and beyond the realm of matter." Two examples of these universal metabolic forces are relaxation and awareness. When applied directly to eating, they are the greatest enhancers of digestion, nutrition, and maintenance of appropriate body weight. That is, when we slow down enough to be fully aware of the food we are eating—taste it, savor it, and make time for relaxation at the dining table—the food nourishes us in ways that no food can when it is wolfed down or gobbled on the run.

Every cell in my body resonated deeply with David's words. I realized that the transubstantial metabolic enhancers he recommends for health, nutrition, and maintenance of optimum weight are undeniably similar to the suggestions I offer couples seeking more satisfying sexual experiences and more loving relationships. These universal metabolic forces and their powerful effects on human sexuality hold absolutely true in my own personal experience. Just as we allow our food to nourish our bodies by eating more slowly, by practicing slow sex we allow our sexual relationships to nourish our bodies, hearts, and souls.

The first step is to change our minds about sex. A shift in perspective opens new doors of experience for the body, giving it space to express itself. Usually our *ideas* about sex are forced onto the body, pushing it to cooperate and fulfill the many expectations and desires we associate with sex. Such pressures have made sex a hurried and single-minded act, whereas the body is inwardly thrilled with a slow, languid, expansive sexual exchange. Rather than *do* so much in sex, the body prefers to *be* in sex. This requires an acute awareness of the present moment. In slow sex, instead of getting involved in building to a climax, you take a step back and witness yourself. You are not so hot; instead you become more cool. Slowness takes the heat out of sex, which is a good thing, because bliss and ecstasy plant their delicate roots in a cool environment, not a hot one.

For the same reason, sexual arousal is not a prerequisite. You don't need to heat up with excitement. Instead, you discover how to fall back into your body, to be more aware and relaxed, with a sense of not really going anywhere special. It doesn't require lots of energy to engage in, or sustain, slow sex. And herein lies one of the main blessings of a slow sex practice—it is a sustainable practice particularly well suited to long-term committed couples. Over a period of many years it is natural for a couple to experience a certain amount of cooling down in sex, because it's simply not possible to stay hot and excited about each other forever. There has to be some maturing, some settling, some turning inward toward resources that lie within yourself, rather than outside of yourself. The nature of heat is that it has to cool down eventually. Coolness is sustainable and it has an eternal quality. This makes slow sex a practice that can grow, deepen, and develop over time. It is a practice that generates love and harmony, creating balance within each person and between two lovers.

This book presents slow sex as a practice for contemporary couples, but it has ancient roots in Eastern spiritual traditions—such as Tantra from India and Taoism from China—that have found expression in a number of current Western sexual movements. Certain Tantric lineages embraced sexual practice to bring about an expansion of consciousness, and as a doorway to the Divine. Taoist inner alchemy practices cultivate sexual energy in order to empower the body and boost health.

"There are very long and rich traditions of sexual mysticism that can be traced back before the origins of Christianity in the West," writes Arthur Versluis in his book *The Secret History of Western Sexual Mysticism,* "and for all the efforts of the 'orthodox' to extirpate it, erotic mysticism still recurs time and again, perpetually renewed, like the phoenix." Versluis believes that sexual mysticism is particularly attractive in the present day and age because it resonates with a deep human need for connection—with another individual, but also to nature and to the Divine. Fulfillment of these needs has eroded in modern Western culture, where disconnection and isolation tend to prevail. I can say with certainty that slow sex is a practice of sexual mysticism that gently heals and restores our isolating severed connections. Sex has a higher potential—sex is able to carry us beyond duality into a spiritual unity that brings us closer to ourselves, the other, nature, and God.

Among the early proponents of contemporary spiritual sexuality was Alice Bunker Stockham, one of the first women to graduate from medical school in the United States, who published a book called *Karezza: Ethics of Marriage* in 1903. Stockham's text states that there is deeper purpose and meaning to the reproductive faculties and functions than is generally understood and taught. She writes about a physical union that can include a joyful soul communion that promotes soul growth and development. So although spirituality in sex may be new to many of us, we can see that sex has been used for higher purposes over and over again in different ways and in very different cultures from ancient times to the present.

Slow sex as a practice leads to a form of spiritual marriage that meets deep human needs for connection and generates a positive rejuvenating energy in a couple, which then spills over into the community. Slow sex represents the only viable way forward for us—as man and woman together—to create a loving and sustainable humanity. It is a powerful way to create peace for ourselves and for the world.

1

SLOW SEX
A Physical and Spiritual Revolution

Slow sex provides a simple and effective antidote to the ever-accelerating pace of modern life, allowing lovers to rest in a still point at the center of a turning world. Through the workshops we offer to couples, my partner and I have been able to see the profound effect that just one week of relaxing slow sex can have on a couple's relationship. We are true believers in the power of taking it slow, but sometimes it appears as if the whole world is bent on spinning faster and faster around us.

That is why it was so thrilling for me to read *The Slow Down Diet* by Marc David. David writes about slowing down in relation to food and I am concerned with slowing down while having sex, but we are really talking about the same thing—the ability to be fully present and aware in the current moment so that we can actually experience life on an inner cellular level, rather than racing through it so quickly that everything flies by in a blur.

David says that for food to be truly nourishing, the invisible "atmospheric" factors—*how* we eat—are even more important than the physical substances we actually consume. I have already mentioned two of the eight universal metabolic enhancers that he defines—relaxation and awareness. The other six are quality, rhythm, pleasure, thought, the sacred, and the story.

In essence, and in my own way, my teaching conveys the need to incorporate these great universal metabolic enhancers into the sexual act, organically elevating the physical exchange into something spiritual and fulfilling. I have also observed that the satisfaction of slow sex acts as a nutrient that boosts the immune system, with rejuvenating effects that increase vitality, creativity, and love. At the same time, slow sex naturally reduces the emphasis on food and eating because we find nourishment and fulfillment elsewhere. It naturally supports weight loss and brings balance into the system, not through vigorous calorie-burning sex, but through extended, deeply satisfying, sensitive sex.

I suggest, for instance, that couples incorporate relaxation and awareness into the sexual act. These two simple "Love Keys" (as I call these universal metabolic enhancers) can greatly transform the sexual experience from a perhaps short-lived and repetitive event into a captivating, extended, and inspiring one. When a couple embraces the universal metabolic enhancers, doing so creates a rarified atmosphere that strengthens and amplifies the field of love surrounding them. In an environment such as this, an inner radiance and vitality will remain as an afterglow.

Such expanded dimensions can even open up when only one person introduces metabolic enhancers into the atmosphere. Just as a sensitive person in the presence of a genuinely spiritual individual may experience a type of transmitted phenomenon that ignites feelings of being more open, alive, expanded, and present, when one person slows down in sex, the second person is naturally drawn into the expanded energy field and will tune in to and link up with the universal metabolizers. The slower we can learn to be, the more we can relax and hold awareness of the present moment; gradually the practice of slowness will begin to positively impact every aspect of living.

The conventional definition of metabolism implies it is a purely physical function, "the sum total of all the chemical reactions in the body." Marc David's understanding goes beyond that, defining metabolism as "the sum total of all the chemical reactions in the body, plus the sum total of all our thoughts, feelings, beliefs, and experiences" (*The Slow Down Diet,* page 8).

David believes that these metabolizers have been in existence for a long time but have been completely overlooked because:

First, we've been moving too fast to notice them, since their chemical power is activated only when the requisite level of "slowness" has been met. Second, we've believed that a metabolic enhancer must be exclusively of the order of a food, a pill, or a push-up, yet the eight universal metabolizers are of a different category. (*The Slow Down Diet,* page 9)

As a professional nutritionist and expert in the psychology of eating, Marc David has applied these universal metabolic insights to people who seek his guidance for nutritional and weight issues. He observed their responses to his unusual dietary suggestions and noted the undeniably positive impact on the entire system. He writes:

The bottom line was this: These folks achieved more by doing less. The people I'm speaking of stopped fighting food and started embracing it. . . . They ceased being victimized by food, by their bodies, and by anyone else's standards and instead took responsibility for making simple but profound changes that created an empowered metabolic state. They slowed down and trusted life. (*The Slow Down Diet,* page 11)

I can say exactly the same thing about the couples who have attended our slow sex workshops. When couples learn to relax into the present moment while having sex, their entire experience is transformed into something deeply touching and nourishing for body and being. The entire metabolism is profoundly influenced and empowered. Because the eight universal metabolic enhancers defined by David apply just as directly to our sexuality as they do to our physical nutrition, I have decided to organize the book around them, just as he has done in *The Slow Down Diet*.

As a way of approaching slow sex, each of the eight universal metabolic enhancers will appear as the focus of a separate chapter. Each chapter will act as an umbrella covering relevant information and guidelines. At times it will be necessary to repeat some information as the sexual themes intertwine and form a bigger picture.

Chapter 2, "The Sexual Power of Relaxation," focuses on relaxing away from *doing* and into simply *being* while having sex—away from goal-oriented sex that strives toward the climax of orgasm, and toward sex that allows things to evolve of their own accord.

Chapter 3, "The Sexual Power of Awareness," focuses on awareness as the missing link to expressing our higher sexual potential. Through awareness we awaken to the body on an inner level and tune in to our intrinsic sexual vitality.

Chapter 4, "The Sexual Power of Quality," focuses on the sexual intelligence lying within our human bodies. It recognizes the fact that our genitals have an innate wisdom about how to connect when we give them the chance and space to communicate in their own language.

Chapter 5, "The Sexual Power of Rhythm," focuses primarily on the difference between male and female rhythms. These polarity differences are understood as complementary forces that can be embraced to bring sex to a higher level of expression.

Chapter 6, "The Sexual Power of Pleasure," focuses on the need for a shift from sensation to sensitivity. Slowness increases sensitivity and trust in the body, and activates the metabolic power of pleasure.

Chapter 7, "The Sexual Power of Thought," focuses on the capacity to think and fantasize, and how these can act as distractions. However, thought can also be used in positive ways that will stimulate the sexual metabolism.

Chapter 8, "The Sexual Power of the Sacred," focuses on sensitivity and coolness as the bridge to divine ecstatic experiences. It explains the healing and purifying power of the genitals.

Chapter 9, "The Sexual Power of the Story," focuses on the inherent human aspects of sex and the historical personal aspects, as well as evaluating slow sex as a step in human evolution.

Each of these is a key to transforming your sex life, often in ways that feel surprisingly easy and natural. As you read each chapter, any insights or curiosities that are stimulated in you as a consequence can be put immediately into practice when you are next with your partner. You need to bear in mind that it's not *what* you do, but *how* you do it, so in that sense it's easy to make subtle changes with little effort. Naturally it's impossible to incorporate all the different aspects at once and expect to get it right the very first time you try slow sex. Sometimes people take to the new way very easily, as if it were second nature, but this tends to be more the exception than the rule.

In a more sensitive society, the opposite would be true—slow sex would be the rule, not the exception. However, we have fundamental misconceptions about sex that act as a barrier to a simple, innocent, and spiritual sexual experience. Because sex has been practiced and presented in a certain way, generation upon generation, it is helpful to have an awareness of our collective conditioning, along with patience and compassion for yourself and your partner. Don't expect instant results! It's more of an unfolding based on exploration and discovery. You become a pioneer of your inner world. You simply start from where you are today—misunderstandings included. To an extent you undergo a process of unlearning what we've all inherited and rediscovering what is real and true. Each time you and your partner get together you will continue to make small exploratory steps, experimenting, incorporating what you discovered (or learned) the previous time, and gradually developing a new sexual language together.

At the end of some chapters, sensitivity and awareness exercises are suggested as a way to tune in to, support, and enhance the cellular perception of the body. The final chapter, chapter 10, "Your Personal Slow Sex Practice," will pull together all of the previous information, offering basic suggestions on how to get started with your own personal practice.

This book is not a technical manual in the sense of being focused on *what you do;* rather, the approach is one of exploring *how you do it.* Much information on "how to proceed" and how to create the atmosphere necessary for an uplifting experience is embedded in the chapters ahead. As you read, you may perhaps begin to notice a subtle shift in the way you view and understand sex. And as I see it, this is the way to go—first and foremost, a change of mind is required. We need a new vision of sex that brings about a change or revolution in our ideas. When there is a change in the mind, the body will easily and willingly respond.

Whenever I get into the details of sex I will often begin by apologizing, because I tend to talk in generalizations that have the effect of bringing us all onto much the same level. As if we are all afloat in the same sexual boat. However, each one of us has an individual personal experience and sexual history, so it is likely that *not* everything I say will hold true for each person. If something does not ring true for you, it means only that it is not true for you as an individual, not that what is said is false; because *generally* speaking, what is said about sex is true. As an overall invitation, please feel free to discard anything that does not ring true for you. And at the same time, be open to something you may have *thought* is not true for you, as well as being interested in what is true for others.

Whether we like it or not, our sexuality affects our total being. Each of us feels the impact of sex from the moment of arrival on Earth in a human body, even if our adult lives may ultimately include rare or no sexual interactions with another person. The conventional and accepted speedy way we have sex circumscribes and reduces our experience of living in our extraordinarily beautiful human bodies. Slow sex enables us to physically and consciously create love and happiness, nourishing us on extremely profound and life-changing levels.

2

THE SEXUAL POWER
OF RELAXATION

M any of us are under the mistaken impression that relaxation
is some kind of floppy, collapsed, and more-or-less dead state.
This is definitely not true. Deep relaxation brings about a state of inner
aliveness and vitality. The real by-product of relaxation is a sense of
regeneration, of feeling refreshed and uplifted.

THE BREVITY OF THE SEX ACT

Humans are living not only longer, but faster. We seem to be speeding
up by the day and by the decade. The stress levels that accompany all
this speed are acute and cumulative, and penetrate deeply into many
aspects of our lives, including our sex lives. Generally speaking, sex
often is, and has always been, a speedy and short-lived event. If what we
see in the movies and what we know from our own sexual experiences
is anything to go by, then sex is mostly comprised of fleeting encounters
of the "wham, bam, thank you, ma'am!" variety.

At present the universal average time of a sexual encounter is estimated to be anywhere from two to three minutes—a time span of 120
to 180 seconds out of a day in which we live through 86,400 seconds.

These "quickies" seem to serve one main purpose, and that is (for the man especially) to have an orgasm as quickly as possible.

Reaching orgasm means that sex is usually finished shortly after it starts. The perhaps much longed-for, or much fantasized, event is compressed into an astoundingly brief period of time. As humans we seem to mimic the animals around us, who are very efficient in their reproduction. They get the job over and done at high speed, because there is usually only one chance, and it's now. But as humans we are granted the privilege of choice. We can engage in sex at any time of the day, week, or year, because we are not restricted to hormonally dictated mating seasons. So why do humans tend to want to get sex over with so quickly, particularly when we have more options in the matter than our animal friends? And then, even with the privilege of choice, strangely enough it often happens that we continually have the urge for the same thing, over and over. It's as if we are caught in a cycle of unfulfilled sexual desire—longing for it, getting it, but only as a temporary measure. Soon the urge or desire will arise again, but satisfying it doesn't seem to leave us in a state of peace and contentment.

Seldom does one hear about a sexual engagement that is consciously extended, hour upon hour. My first really long lovemaking experience was thirteen hours nonstop, from dusk to dawn. At that point I had been more accustomed to five or six hours at a time. And then, at some time further on in my exploration, my new lover and I were in bed for a solid twenty-one days, apart from the minimum of time required to care for bodily needs. We ate only occasionally, finding ourselves satiated by something other than food. We were "in" love, constantly fused in an ecstatic state of timelessness and rapture, suspended in a miraculous web of the unfolding moment. We did not sleep, as we had no need of it. Night merged with day, day with night, in one continuum of sexual presence, passion, and spontaneity, literally tapped into an awesome, abundant source of life.

Some people experience similar remarkable exchanges and interactions of a higher frequency, but invariably these connections happen spontaneously, and are likely to be relatively isolated. Usually a person is unable to consciously create similar experiences on a sustained basis as a style of sexual expression.

The Tedium of Repetition

Even though there is certainly pleasure to be had in sexual quickies, the experience is essentially brief and there is simply not enough time for anything exotic or extraordinary to happen between two bodies. Bodies are similar to musical instruments, and usually need to first be tuned individually. Then they need time to warm up and attune to each other. Only then is it possible for the sounds to dance together in the creation of a musically engaging piece. But usually, where the musical creativity of sex is concerned, many people will admit that the experience can be repetitive and a little bit boring (unless we change partners to spice things up). The repetition is not inherent to sex itself, but occurs because we are sticking to certain sexual habits and patterns. In some cases it's even an addiction—doing more or less the same thing, year in and year out. We don't really know how to bring variety and creativity into our sexual encounters. The full spectrum of human sexual experience allows us to consciously choose to make a fundamental shift in our sexual ways. When we are able to transcend our habits and patterns, we are easily able to generate and make love in the way we were designed by the Divine. Through engaging in a more informed style of sexual interaction we are able to create love, joy, and sustenance for ourselves.

RELAXATION IS VITAL
FOR THE SEXUAL METABOLISM

The way forward for us as humans is to engage in sex with increasing ease, leisure, and relaxation. In taking speed and stress out of the sexual act, we remove the performance pressure that comes with filling expectations and achieving goals. We allow time and space for the experience, in the sense of being able to extend the meeting as a matter of choice. A slow approach in sex acts like a "medicine" that is easily able to resolve and heal many long-term sexual problems and wounds that cause unhappiness, separation, and insecurity. The majority of our problems can be reduced to our sexual problems, so it is obvious that we need to make some changes.

Being, Rather than Doing

Relaxation is generally something we afford ourselves only when most of our daily tasks are done. Trying to fit everything into our busy schedules frequently creates time-management stress, and we give little value to the benefits of sheer relaxation and the joy of doing nothing. When the endless list is more or less complete, only then do we grant ourselves permission to take a break. Often by this stage we fall into an exhausted sleep or drift off into a doze. Perhaps we read a book or watch television. These moments definitely represent time off, but they don't amount to true relaxation, which is highly refreshing in its effects.

Many of us afford ourselves very little in the way of relaxation because we believe that to be "doing" something has intrinsic value. In fact, we sometimes feel that we are doing something wrong or feel guilty if we are doing, literally, nothing. Simply relaxing into a space of being, or non-doing, is judged by ourselves, and perhaps by others, as laziness or a lack of ambition and goals. We don't approve of that in our speed- and goal-driven culture.

THE GOAL OF ORGASM INTERFERES WITH RELAXATION

Relaxation becomes a challenge when we have survival stress and anxiety compounded by many different goals to achieve, and dreams and expectations to fulfill. Sex, likewise, is filled to the brim with goals and expectations. We enter sex with an agenda, with a clear sense of knowing exactly what we want or expect. Then we set about engineering these desired results with intention and tension. We base our approach on previous experiences, which are, in turn, rooted in conventional ideas about sex that we unconsciously inherit from our society.

In sex it is not common to simply relax and enjoy what is happening in the moment, waiting to see where our bodies want to take us, allowing things to evolve of their own accord. Our desire to have an orgasm, or "come," is often why most of us want sex in the first place. Having the goal of orgasm causes stress about performance and satisfaction, so we rush toward the finish to make sure we get there. We get ahead of the body and use the body, pushing it, forcing it to obey and follow the mind's instructions. However, the pressure and tension we bring into the situation has the ultimate and actual effect of making us less sensitive. The sheer speed of it all deadens us to the vitality and inner aliveness streaming through our human flesh. Being distracted by an anticipated orgasm and working toward building to a climax literally prevents us from being rooted in the body, from being in the here and now, connected to the actual moment-by-moment experience of the body.

Having orgasm as a goal causes a kind of absence because the focus lies slightly ahead of where we actually are. It make us always more interested in the *next* penetration, and not particularly interested in *this* one, because the next one will bring us closer to the desired goal, to the climax. In being one step ahead of ourselves, we miss the pure joy of devoting total attention to each glorious penetration, man giving and woman receiving in perfect communion. When we can be more still in mind and body, we can listen to our inner wisdom and and honor the natural ways of the body. Slowing down and relaxing away from goals will open up a new window of sexual experience to explore. Finding full value in sex, pursuing its human aspects and its great potential, lies beyond the boundaries of the common quickie.

Premature Ejaculation

Man has an easier time than woman in the quickie approach, in that sex is usually over when the man ejaculates. Often the man will finish well before the woman has sufficiently warmed up to the experience.

For the majority of women, reaching an orgasm within a few minutes of penetration is not so easy. Ten, fifteen, or twenty minutes are not necessarily enough either. Women will often require additional stimulation of the clitoris in order to reach a climax. Yet the majority of men are not really able to hold back their ejaculation in order to intentionally extend lovemaking. Ejaculation will usually be experienced as an overwhelming wave, impossible to stop or sidestep. It takes control of the body, somewhat like a sneeze that suddenly emerges from nowhere and takes you over. To intentionally refrain from ejaculation, a man must from time to time relax back into his body and take several deep breaths. These pauses take the focus off increasing the excitement and help to bring more attention to the body in the present moment. As soon as orgasm as the goal of sex is dropped, relaxation into the present follows naturally.

The underlying reason for a man's premature ejaculation is too much stress and tension, particularly in the form of sexual stimulation and excitement, which (as we will explore in later chapters) has little to do with pure pleasure and ecstasy. There are also many psychological stresses that create tension and contraction in the system, such as performance pressure and wanting to be successful, fear of not being good enough, fear of coming too soon, wanting to satisfy and please, ego desire to be this particular woman's best lover ever, and so on. With relaxation, ejaculation can easily be postponed. The effort and stimulation necessary to achieve orgasm falls away, with the result that the whole system relaxes and the body is then able to be more present. If you want to avoid premature ejaculation, then drop the idea that orgasm is central to sex. Slowing down movements will automatically reduce the level of excitement, which is a good thing; it's what we want. Even if a man has suffered from untimely ejaculation all his life, miracles are definitely possible when a relaxed sexual attitude is adopted. One man shared during a couples retreat several years ago that he had been able to overcome a thirty-year premature ejaculation problem *overnight,* simply by monitoring and reducing his level of excitement.

The suggestion to reduce the level of excitement holds true for women, too. If a woman wishes to make love for longer periods of time, she should reduce movements that cause stimulation and excitement, instead holding still at times, poised and present. One particularly good reason for a woman to avoid high levels of stimulation is that her excitement is frequently the trigger for a man's early ejaculation. Fortunately, it is well within a woman's power to relax back into herself and thereby postpone her partner's ejaculation. Instead of going for an orgasm, she creates a situation that is inviting and welcoming, without being exciting. Remaining in the cooler zone of sexual experience will naturally keep a man's ejaculation at bay.

The Containment of Semen Empowers Man

One tablespoon of semen is incredibly powerful stuff, almost atomic in its potency. In addition to sperm cells, seminal fluid contains an immense amount of protein, vitamins, minerals, and amino acids, as well as vital energies. Semen contained within the male body represents tremendous individual potential and creative power. It should really be viewed as a type of liquid gold, and not taken so lightly. Dispersed semen represents a loss of personal energy resources, particularly when a man's climax involves the buildup of much tension and stress that leave behind traces in the body, brain chemistry, and psyche. The vast majority of men will admit that after an orgasm they feel depleted, low in energy, disconnected, or withdrawn. Containment of semen will empower a man because the vital substances nourish his intelligence and creativity; he becomes more centered and master of himself.

Relaxation happens easily when we change the idea that orgasm has to happen as a necessary part of sex. When we take away the goal or intention of orgasm, there is no need for a push toward the finish line. With nowhere to go there is no hurry, so everything can unfold in a unique organic way. There is no need to force the body along a certain direction because the body's innate intelligence has other plans in store for us.

DEEP SLOW BREATHING
INVITES RELAXATION

Relaxation is supported through deep slow breathing, because breath brings an infusion of vitality to the system. Deep slow breathing causes an increase in the release of endorphins—neurochemicals produced by the body that act like opiates—into the system, which helps to produce relaxation and a sense of well-being. When we neglect to pay attention to our breath, it often remains only in the chest and shoulders. It's beneficial to invite the breath downward through the diaphragm and into the belly, allowing the belly to rise and fall with the in-breaths and out-breaths. And if you wish you can imagine, or with practice perhaps even feel, that the breath is able to internally caress the genital area.

Conscious breathing in the direction of the genitals during sex increases the oxygen intake and enhances the whole metabolism, providing you with sexual vitality and aliveness. Throughout lovemaking, simply paying acute attention to the process of the in-breaths and the out-breaths can shift you to another realm of experience. Normally breathing is involuntary and happens whether we're thinking about it or not, which makes it extremely easy to slip out of conscious connection with the breath. It is a function of the autonomic nervous system, meaning that its function is independent of the conscious mind. We are not able to consciously affect most processes of our autonomic nervous system, but we can take an active part in our breathing process. The extent to which you relax and deepen the breath as you make love will definitely pay off with the rewards of greater presence, enhanced cellular sensitivity, and inner expansion.

Some people like to make a little ritual of taking several deep slow breaths before actually doing anything. For instance, before you start the ignition of your car, stop, take a couple of breaths as you relax your shoulders. Or, when practicing slow sex, take a couple of conscious breaths and become centered in your body for a few moments before you hug your partner. And again, take several breaths before you bring your lips together in a sealed kiss, repeatedly using breath to relax and prepare you for any meeting and exchange. The same thing can be done when a man poises with his penis at the entrance to the vagina, immediately prior to actual penetration. And then once inside, stopping frequently for a couple of deep breaths along the way. The penis can travel breath by breath and fraction by fraction into the vagina, and this journey into woman's body can last for many pleasurable minutes. Once fully inside, a man can remain within the depths, alert and breathing consciously for an extended period of time.

When you touch your partner's body, hold your hands still and give your partner your full inner attention as you take a few breaths into your belly or genitals. Or breathe deeply and consciously as you slowly caress your partner's body with a feather-light touch. Avoid any kind of stimulation that will trigger the desire for orgasm, which can easily leave us a bit breathless. Or at least take a few breathing breaks between bouts of excitement. A little excitement, then relax and breathe; then a little more excitement, and again relax. Whenever you find yourself focusing on the next penetration and eventual orgasm, if you stop all movement and be still for a while, taking a few deep breaths, it will help you to cool down and relax into the here and now.

LINING UP THE BONES

I have found that the depth of relaxation depends substantially on the physical body position; literally, how the bones line up as a skeleton. Relaxation requires a certain physical poise, which means physical alignment, and alignment brings presence to a body and grace to movement. A certain tension level is required to hold most upright sitting positions, and tension is part of our physical integrity, but any extra or habitual tension can be consciously released. The body will usually respond to this conscious letting go and relaxation of tensions with a spontaneous deep breath in gratitude.

CREATE TIME FOR SEX

It is much easier to be relaxed about sex when you grant yourself adequate space and time for the sexual exchange. To support relaxation you can actually make an appointment with your partner for sex, in the same way that you make time for meals, work, the gym, friends, and children. Set aside enough time and space to allow yourselves to warm up and physically attune to each other. Decide together on the time and place for the experience.

Exercises: Daily Observation and Conscious Relaxation Practices

↺ Scanning from Head to Toe for Tension

You can do this simple practice at any time of the day and in almost any place. The body gets tense and a bit contracted without our realizing it, and this type of tension has a compressing effect on your body energy during daily life, which also carries over into sex. The body carries many subtle and not-so-subtle tensions. As you make love (or sit, walk, drive, and so on), repeatedly scan your body from head to toe, or toe to head, and deliberately and consciously relax any areas of tension that you encounter. The following are some classic places where we hold tension without realizing it:

- Around the mouth
- In the joints of the jaw (the temporomandibular joint, or TMJ)
- In the neck and shoulders
- In the solar plexus (the soft spot below the upside-down V formed by the rib cage)
- In the belly
- In the feet

↺ Relaxing the Pelvic Floor

Another central and significant place to consciously relax is the pelvic floor, which means the web of muscles and tissues that surround the anus and genitals. Invariably this muscular floor will be slightly contracted and pulled upward, without our being aware of this tension. Let go of any tightness you discover there, and do so a hundred times during the day or whenever you happen to remember. Intentionally relaxing and releasing any subtle holding and tension in the muscles will allow the pelvic floor to widen and drop slightly.

- For a woman, relaxing the pelvic floor means taking the attention to the vagina and relaxing any tightness or holding discovered there.
- For a man it means consciously relaxing and letting go of the anus and the muscles of the buttocks.

To feel the difference between tension and then relaxation, you can first exaggerate the tension, and then release it. Tighten genitals and anus, pulling upward and inward, hold for a few seconds, and then release slowly.

Make Conscious Relaxation an Everyday Practice

Invariably, as soon as our attention has moved away from the part we have consciously relaxed, the tension gradually begins to return and assert itself. So scanning the body from head to toe and relaxing tensions can be done intermittently. We will probably never completely rid ourselves of these subtle tensions, and that is really not the aim or goal. The aim is to remember that you are first and foremost a body—and to notice when and where you are tense, and then to intentionally relax these tense parts. Let go, take a deep breath, and feel your body. This little process is something to be done billions of times, not just once or twice. Relaxation of different body parts creates inner space and expansion and is usually followed by a wave of sensitivity on a delicate cellular level.

There are myriad small, insignificant daily actions in which we can practice conscious relaxation: brushing our teeth, washing dishes, preparing food, driving, opening and closing doors, sitting at the computer, and standing in line at the bank or checkout, to name but a few. Paying attention to your level of relaxation during the day will support your experience in bed, and vice versa.

3

THE SEXUAL POWER OF AWARENESS

If you have tried scanning your body and relaxing any tense areas that you notice, that in itself was an act of awareness. So if you are not sure what awareness means, and you managed to relax your jaw, shoulders, and belly, you are already using that particular witnessing power or aptitude. Awareness is not far away from us, and indeed, we would not be able to survive without a certain level of awareness. At the same time, we know remarkably little about the power of awareness and how it can change our every moment.

AWARENESS IS THE MISSING LINK

For human beings, awareness during sex is the missing link to expressing and living our higher sexual potential. This uniquely human capacity to observe ourselves as if from a distance has a tremendously powerful impact on metabolism and sexual responsiveness. Awareness acts as a highly potent aphrodisiac. Through awareness we awaken to the body on an inner level and tune in to our intrinsic, God-given sexual vitality. Awareness is the capacity to observe and witness oneself—as a body and as a mind filled with the thoughts that distance us from the body—in any given moment of any given day, including, of course, while we are having sex. As Marc David notes:

> One of the most unusual scientific revelations of the last century is the mathematical proof that the act of observing any phenomenon in the universe—be it the flight of a bird or the rotation of a planet— has a direct influence upon that phenomenon. According to the laws of physics, we have no choice but to alter the bird's course or the planet's speed simply by focusing our awareness on it. So if we have the power to tweak the orbit of a heavenly body, it should come as no surprise that vitamin A—awareness—also has a profound impact on the human body. (*The Slow Down Diet,* page 62)

Awareness is the driving force behind slow sex. As we become intensely aware of each and every breath, touch, movement, or shift of the body, the sexual experience unfolds and flows easily and effortlessly moment by moment. And if we so wish, the exchange can continue for hours on end according to, and being guided by, what wants to happen between the bodies themselves. For extended lovemaking there needs to be no agenda, no goal, just an appreciation of the here-and-now experience. So to some extent you are faced with dropping the ego and the sexual personality with its demands, likes and dislikes, habits and addictions. Slowness is basic to a shift in sexual experience—slowing down in all you do, giving yourself the space to tune in to yourself. Be slow in your approach to the other person as well, and above all be slow, easy, and relaxed as you join your bodies and become one.

Relaxation and awareness actually go hand in hand, because you have to become more aware of your physical body in order to release any tension, clenching, tightness, or holding. Awareness, therefore, precedes relaxation, and relaxation in turn deepens the awareness. When you consciously relax you will usually feel an inner wave of vitality, light, or aliveness expanding through the body. The delight of these inner sensations in turn engages the awareness, enabling you to fall into even deeper relaxation.

Once we find our way into the intangible present through awareness, we develop the qualities and radiance of true "presence." Awareness
is the capacity to be alert to what *is*. It's the ability to be in touch with
what is happening inside you and around you this very moment. When
we build awareness into our sexual expression, it is the most powerful
metabolic force.

IT'S NOT WHAT YOU DO
BUT HOW YOU DO IT

As we explore further we will discover that it is well-nigh impossible to
make rules about how to be slow. Creating a shift in our sexual experience is definitely not about following a set of rules; it's more of an inquiry.
It's an ongoing effort to feel yourself and be self-observant during sex. It is
examining not only what you are doing, but more importantly, how you
are doing it. We simply do whatever we do as consciously as possible, with
all the alertness we can muster in any given moment.

We usually say in our workshops that when you are making love,
everything and anything goes, because it's not what you do, but how
you do it. Any act done with awareness is changed by that awareness
itself, so the "what" can be transformed through the "how." In this way
being slow can never be a special sexual technique. It is not something
you can do as such, because slowness is actually an outcome or by-
product of what happens when an action is carried out with awareness.

You may already have discovered how difficult it is to *do* slow, especially when accustomed to a faster approach. Most of us have had the
experience of driving along in a car, totally engaged in the movement
and momentum, when all of a sudden a road sign saying "Slow" or
"Stop" appears. At such a point, being forced to go slowly is a disturbance that can lead to irritation and frustration. Imagine, then, during
sex when you are in full swing and then unexpectedly you remember the
suggestion to go slow. Or you have it fixed in your mind that you have
to be slow because you have been instructed to be slow. With this kind

of rule-oriented attitude, the exploration of slowness will be tedious, not easy. In fact being slow will probably be the last thing you feel like doing when in the throes of a sexual encounter. The mind likes to do things right and stick with the rules, but this lack of flexibility closes the door to exploration. An inquiry requires curiosity, alertness, and a willingness to step into the unknown.

BEING CONSCIOUS
INSTEAD OF MECHANICAL

The bottom-line truth is that most of the time we humans are not fully present in, or aware in, our beautifully sensitive fleshy bodies. We are not really connected to them on an inner level. We habitually use them in mechanical ways and do not really pay attention during most of our activities, except when physical pain is experienced. We remember the spine when we unexpectedly have a backache or the knee only when it hurts every time we bend it. Over time, especially as our bodies begin to show signs of wear and tear, our associations with the body can become negative and draining, not positive, nourishing, and uplifting.

Seldom do we focus ourselves sufficiently to consciously experience the actual "how" of what we are doing. Because we do the same things again and again, there is a mechanization in the way we conduct our daily activities—walk, sit, stand, lie down, drive, cook, clean, shower, shave, shampoo, or whatever. We don't use our awareness. How are you sitting right now, as you are reading, for instance? Where is your body and how is your spine, your head, your neck? Collapsed forward or in one connected line? Shoulders up or down? Jaw clenched or relaxed? Breathing? When did you last consciously feel your breath? Are you holding your breath or is it shallow? Enjoy a deep breath right now!

As we get busy dealing with the demands of the day, our focus is, for the most part, outside of the body. Our attention is on achievement, getting something done, but not on the physical process involved in getting there. We lack a certain presence in all of our activities, including, of course, sex. We all have personal goals and doggedly set off each time in a mechanical, driven way in an attempt to reach a pleasing end. And as mentioned before, satisfying our immediate desires causes us to be absent, marginally present to the moment, ourselves, the other.

USE AWARENESS
TO REMAIN IN THE NOW

As your level of awareness grows, everything becomes slower and more deliberate, creating an opportunity to feel and follow the wisdom and intelligence residing within the human body. A change in sexual experience becomes possible with the insight that the goal or habit of orgasm acts as a temptation in the future (see previous chapter), seducing us away from an awareness of the simple, authentic here and now.

Imagine for a moment that you have been used to spinning happily along in an automatic car and then unexpectedly you have to adjust to a less familiar manual shift. With a manual shift, gears are changed by hand in a more sequenced step-by-step way, coordinating with the clutch and engine speed. More awareness is needed, naturally, especially in the beginning when it is quite easy to stall the car. You are required to pay attention to the engine, tune in to its sounds, listen to the engine revolutions until they reach the right pitch, then do some speedy fancy footwork to release the gas, press the clutch, shift the gear with your hand, then release the clutch, and reapply pressure to the accelerator, all in one flowing move. These shifts are repeated again and again depending on traffic density or the road's curves, shifting gears down and up again. At first this kind of deliberate driving is bound to feel awkward and unfamiliar, and to get it right takes practice, but before long it becomes an integral part of driving. Eventually the moves will flow smoothly, but maintaining attention to the sound of the engine is an ongoing process.

We can change our patterns of lovemaking in much the same way. Instead of accelerating immediately to top gear, we can consciously cause a change in the course of events by choosing to become more aware of each shift in the situation. And the transition begins with *not* running after something, which makes it simpler. We do not fast-forward directly toward orgasm. Deliberately and with intention we stay here, remaining present. We already have some kind of awareness of the components required to pull an orgasm together, so to create the opposite and not dash forward must be an option as well. When we withdraw from fantasy or stimulation or anything that puts pressure on or inflames the situation, we forestall the urge that so easily becomes a compulsion. We no longer feel forced to give in to the pressing urgency to climax and release.

Open Eyes Increase Awareness

Our eyes are tools that put us in direct contact with our immediate surroundings in the present. Often sex takes place with closed eyes and in the dark, and usually sexual fantasy involves closed eyes, but during slow sex you can begin to experiment with keeping them open and receptive. You can begin to make a practice of receiving with your eyes when you are looking at nature, imagining that nature is looking back at you. You reverse the perspective of vision. You are not looking out, but are being looked into by the other. This can be done with a tree, a flower, a bird, a beautiful sunset, the moon, stars, snowcapped peaks, a waterfall, the sunrise, or any lovely creation of nature, including another human being. The eyes can just be open, receiving, and inviting. (See the soft vision exercise at the end of this chapter.)

With the eyes open, staying in awareness, we naturally slow down to the extent that the usual triggers for climax are minimized. Sounds like contrary sexual advice, doesn't it? Usually the recommendation would be to maximize whatever brings us to a peak, but here we are placing attention on a critical point. We want to gently simmer and not boil over. We are monitoring ourselves—noticing what we are doing and how we are doing it—by engaging our awareness.

ENERGY FOLLOWS ATTENTION

Direct your awareness to your own body during lovemaking. You take the focus away from your partner's body and direct it inwardly toward yourself. As you relax and remain present to what is, you become better able to actually feel what is happening in your own body. Instead of attention being focused on orgasm or the other, you have the opportunity and space to turn inward and connect to your inner world at the outset.

The physical body ought to be given primary place in your field of awareness. When you focus on being rather than on doing, you can now bring attention, using your inner eye, to a flesh and bone level. And here you uncover new realms, a cosmos of cellular aliveness and vitality that is the domain of the invisible inner body. Uniting with the inner world makes a world of difference to your experience of sex, because you enter the domain of your awe-inspiring senses.

Allowing your awareness to penetrate the body tissues brings you alive to your embodied self. Love is made with and between bodies, and the body acts as an anchor to the present—a simple bridge to the inner qualities of sensitivity, being, and love.

Shifting focus from outer stimuli to the sensitivity of the inner body requires some practice, which means it may take time to get the knack of feeling yourself from another perspective. It's no big deal, really; instead of the more familiar "up and out," where the attention is focused outside yourself, you draw back and pull your attention into your own body. Simple. Your attention becomes free to move inward, and you will observe that if you put your attention on any pleasing inner experience, that sensitivity, energy, vitality, aliveness, chi, prana, or life force (call it what you will) actually increases. That's the power of awareness. Any sensations of streaming, tingling, vibrating, or warmth, for instance, will respond to the awareness and amplify, expanding deliciously into other parts of the body.

In *The Slow Down Diet* I found confirmation of this thrilling inner phenomenon:

In the yoga tradition there's a saying that has helped practitioners reach for greater levels of mastery in working with the body: "Where attention goes, energy flows." Decades of research in biofeedback have certainly proved this axiom, for when we focus on most any area of the body we can increase blood flow, alter bioelectric potential, and influence the secretion of numerous biochemicals. (*The Slow Down Diet,* page 75)

In other words, all these physiological responses to awareness create pleasurable, engaging, sensitive subtle sensations within the body. These experiences are touching and fulfilling; they make you feel better about yourself, improving your sense of self-worth and dignity. With awareness you can set out on a journey into the abundant delights and thrills of relaxation. As you become more aware, you relax more. And the more you relax, the more your awareness increases. With more awareness, relaxation can deepen even further. And so it goes, ad infinitum. The forces of the universal metabolic enhancers complement and weave together in a magical, mysterious, consciousness-enhancing way.

COME HOME TO YOURSELF

The fundamental step to developing awareness is to come back to yourself. In order to shift your attention "in and down," rather than "up and out," begin by making the effort of being more aware of your body, noticing how it feels and where it feels. As suggested earlier, sometimes it's easier to become more aware of tensions if you first tighten and deliberately exaggerate the level of tension. Contract and tighten your upper body for a few seconds, and then suddenly let go in one instant, releasing and relaxing all the muscles of the shoulders, jaw, belly, arms, and hands. Your body will take a beautifully deep breath and you will easily be able to feel the subtle pleasure and delight of relaxation course though your body in waves. In the same way, you can consciously (not mechanically) contract and relax the pelvic floor to increase your inner awareness and enhance the vitality of the area. If you wish you can contract on an in-breath to the count of four or five, and then relax on the out-breath to the same number of counts.

Returning to your body requires that you invert your attention on yourself. If you continue to scan your body throughout the day, making it a daily practice to do everything with as much physical awareness and relaxation as you can manage, you will become immersed in your body and develop a natural sensual grace and slowness.

Remember to honor yourself first; your inner connection to your own body is more significant than any connection to your partner's body. It may sound confusing to hear that you and your body are the priority, and not your partner, but this rerouting of attention will help both of you to be alive to yourselves right from the outset. Focusing too much on the other person would be like leaving home, abandoning your own fire tending, and instead going to ignite somebody else's fire to warm that person's house.

When you honor yourself first, you stoke your own fire. You don't depend on someone else to do it for you, and neither does your partner. The two individual fires join, they augment and enhance each other, and fueled by awareness, flames rise in splendid unison.

When our attention is split, partly on the other and partly on ourselves, we disempower ourselves by reducing our sexual potential. The simple act of attending to two or more stimuli at once can dramatically decrease the sexual metabolism. In sex there is a need to focus on yourself first and foremost to boost the fire of your own sexual metabolism.

Exercise: Going In and Down to Find Home in the Body

☉ Identifying an Inner Center of Deep Relaxation

You can do this exercise right now, wherever and however you are sitting in this moment. Or experiment with it later when you are lying or standing. It's a simple way to connect to the inner dimensions of the body.

1. Close your eyes gently.

2. Scan your body and relax your shoulders, jaw, belly, or any place where you feel some tension or holding (see suggestions at the end of chapter 2). Take two or three easy, full breaths through the diaphragm and into your belly.

3. Then, with your eyes closed, begin to imagine that your eyes are looking backward into your body. Keep looking backward and use that inner vision to help you draw your attention into the body and then downward, so that you can sense yourself more from the inside.

4. Start to look around for a place inside the body that feels like home to you. A place that connects you to your body, the inner realms of ease, a place you can settle in to, one that makes you feel rested, as if you are arriving at home in yourself.

   Home can be anywhere below the head—spine, buttocks, belly, genitals, heart, breasts, low back, feet, or anywhere that feels good and right to you. Home can also be the entire body.

5. From home, wherever it happpens to be, however big or small, you can begin to spread your attention and link home to other parts that feel good, as if embracing other pleasant cellular sensations. Or you can expand symmetrically outward from the spine as the midline of the body.

An inner home acts as a resting place, a connection point, working like an anchor that roots the awareness within the body.

Exercise: Practicing Soft Vision with Your Partner

☉ Using the Eyes as a Window into Your Being

The practice of being receptive with a tree or some aspect of nature, described earlier in this chapter, can be extended to a very nice practice with your partner.

1. Close your eyes and connect internally, as described in the previous exercise.

2. When you feel rooted within your body, you can begin to open your eyes fraction by fraction (without losing contact with your inner body—if you do lose this connection, please close your eyes again until you inwardly reconnect, then again slowly open).

3. When your eyes are fully open, gently meet your partner's eyes. Allow your partner into you through the eyes. Let your eyes be easy, soft, receptive, and inviting. It's okay to blink, this is not a staring exercise.

4. Gaze receptively at one eye at a time because trying to engage both of your partner's eyes simultaneously has a mesmerizing, unfocused effect. Perhaps you will notice it is easier to connect with your partner's left eye than the right. Or vice versa. Whichever eye feels comfortable for you, stay with it. Shift to the other eye at any time. If you have a vision deficiency, make any adjustments in distance that you need.

5. Take a deep breath into your belly and allow your eyes to receive what is there in front of them, rather than looking outward in an objective or judgmental fashion.

6. Take several deep breaths into your belly. Scan your body for random areas of tension, and relax them. Relax the belly and soften the muscles surrounding the genitals.

7. Enjoy another breath. Be present in your body, simple and easy.

8. Remain in receptive eye sharing mode for as long as it feels comfortable, and close the eyes whenever it feels necessary, either to reestablish an inner connection or as opportunity to sense yourself more deeply on the inside. Keep coming back to open eyes and being available to yourself on the inside as you receive your partner's soft gaze into you. Avoid keeping the eyes closed for extended periods.

9. When it feels appropriate or when there is a spontaneous drawing together of your bodies, move into a sustained embrace in which you can close your eyes; stay present and attentive to inner details as you relax your body and melt with your partner.

4

THE SEXUAL POWER
OF QUALITY

Quality is born when we tune into the sexual intelligence lying within our human bodies. Quality is born when we are aware and relaxed enough to experience the inherent vitality of the sexual organs. Quality is born when we slow down enough to allow the bodies to connect in their own way and at their own pace.

GENITAL INTELLIGENCE

While it may sound a bit strange, the genitals do have an innate wisdom. They know what to do, how to do it, and when to do it, but only when we create the appropriate atmosphere, surrender, and allow them to function on their own terms. When there is an intentional withdrawal from building to a climax, we offer our sexual organs the opportunity and space to communicate in their own language. The genitals have their own way of communing, of sharing and exchanging energy, and it's nothing short of a miracle. The intelligence built into the genitals can best be described as "biomagnetic" or "electromagnetic."

Man and woman are extremely similar on many levels, yet vastly different on others. We experience this divergence in various ways, but how deep does the difference between us really lie? Beyond our differences in gender, physical appearance, and associated reproductive functions, what is the crucial distinction between man and woman?

On a profound energy level, the basic difference between us is one of polarity. A difference in polarity implies a difference in potential, and this polarity, embedded as an inherent capacity, is lodged as a powerful cellular intelligence in the genital tissues. There exists a polarity difference between the penis and the vagina that gives rise to a spontaneous flow of life force, vitality, energy, chi, prana—call it what you will.

MALE DYNAMIC FORCE, FEMALE RECEPTIVE FORCE

In essence, the male force is a dynamic force (but not a doing force), and the female force is receptive (also not a doing force). So in this sense both man and woman need to refrain from too much doing or activity in sex so that they can open to and access their essence. When we relax back into ourselves and become more aware, we come to exist as opposite forces in relation to each other. One organically gives, flows, or channels, as the other receives, takes in, or absorbs.

These equal forces are fundamentally opposite forces. (See chapter 5 for elaboration on this theme.) One is not less and one is not more; they are in perfect balance and harmony. Too easily we think of receptive as passive, floppy, and lifeless, or dynamic as action and accomplishment, but dynamic and receptive are equally powerful. These qualities are states and not something that can be achieved, except by falling back into your body and being to touch your natural essence.

Male and Female Forces Are Complementary

These two forces are equal yet opposite, and that implies that they are deeply complementary. Without one, the other does not exist. The male force is one half, the female force is the other half. Dynamic can only be dynamic, start to become a stream, or flow, when the container is inwardly prepared to receive such emanations. Receptivity is a powerful state of vitality and presence in which true passion is a surrendering to the genius of nature's ways. Without the quality of receptivity there is little chance for man to respond in true male dynamic fashion. In this way man is relatively dependent on the female environment that surrounds his penis, the quality of relaxation, awareness, and receptivity in the vaginal tissues. Similarly, when a man is present and aware in his penis, woman is more easily able to relax into herself, and in so doing, increase the capacity to receive the dynamic force.

"Positive" dynamic and "negative" receptive complement each other, and when joined together, the two forces become one unit, whole and complete. The complementary quality of the male and female poles is understood to be the source of our strong intuitive attraction to the opposite gender. And why sexual union appeals to us, calls us, and draws us.

Everything in existence that is not complete seeks completion. And in sex we find completion between ourselves through joining with the equal and opposite force, merging and melting into one integrated whole. The dynamic and receptive forces of the genitals are elements that cannot be seen, even under a microscope, but can be plainly observed in action.

EMBRACING POLARITY HERALDS A CHANGE IN DIMENSION

When you relax into the polarity level of the inner reality there is a shift to an altered state, to a new dimension where you perceive expansion, space, light, love, beauty, eternity. For such a spontaneous effect to take place, you (as individuals) have to position yourselves both physically and mentally.

I recently gained a fascinating insight into the word *dimension*. I was talking to a friend, sharing my personal observation that when I make very simple physical shifts of body position and adjust my alignment, a space opens up and presence and awareness is amplified. He surprised me by saying that he had fully investigated the ancient Greek, or Hellenic, language derivation of the word *dimension*. *Dimension* is rooted in the Hellenic ΔΙΑΣΤΑΣΙΣ, or *thiastasis*. There are two parts. First, ΔΙΑ (*thia*) which means "through" or "to divide." Second, ΣΤΑΣΙΣ (*stasis*), which comes from the verb ΙΣΤΑΜΑΙ (*istame*), which literally means "to place the body in a posture of stillness." At the same time, *thiastasis* means "the size of something when it is still." And the related *ekstasis* means "what comes out of the body's stillness." Embedded in the language lies the intelligence that position, stillness, and dimension are inseparable. A shift of position is required on two levels—mind and body. If we start with the mind, the body usually follows suit. There needs to be an intention to create a situation in which the complementary qualities of male and female come into play as dynamic and receptive forces, wherein man gives and woman receives. The basic direction of the flow is from man into woman, but the container needs to be in a state of poised receptivity to draw the flow of the dynamic force into itself.

The dynamic and receptive functions of the genitals are very clearly attested to by their physical shapes. Nature is very precise, not at all haphazard. The exterior male genitalia is designed to enter the interior female genitalia, and by virtue of being in the appropriate or "right" position in relation to her, has the capacity to channel vitality into her when she is in a correspondingly appropriate position to receive.

LUBRICATION OF THE GENITALS

To facilitate a slow journey into the vagina, it's recommended to begin with lubrication every time you get together. Apply lubricant generously around the entrance and lips of the vagina, as well as over the entire length and head of the penis. Unscented pure oil is recommended. A pure thin vegetable oil, such as almond oil, works well because a little goes a long way. The sensual slipperiness of oil allows for a silky smooth slow entry that can last several minutes as the vaginal canal is gradually probed open. If more oil is needed it can be added at any time. Sesame oil is used in ayurvedic preparations for the genitals. Olive oil can also be used but is a thicker type of oil, better for emergencies rather than for regular use. Oils that are commercially available will usually have natural fragrances added, however a pure unscented oil is advised. Almond oil is usually available over the counter in drugstores. Commercial synthetic lubricant preparations are not made of natural ingredients and can have side effects, such as clogging the deeper part of the vagina and affecting menstrual flow. Important to remember is that oil should *not* be used in conjunction with condoms; instead use a water-based pharmaceutical gel.

SLOW CONSCIOUS ENTRY

The initial approach and very first entry into woman's body is of great significance in keeping excitement to a low level. How a woman is entered sets the atmosphere or tone and will have a tremendous impact on whatever follows. This applies equally when a woman is having sex for the first time and every time thereafter. When man has an erection (see later section for when he does not), the actual entry and subsequent penetration should be done with extreme awareness, and therefore extreme slowness, extending into the vaginal canal millimeter by millimeter, and the slower the better. He should stop any time he feels resistance in the vaginal tissue, which needs time to warm up to receive and absorb the penis.

There are a variety of positions from which to begin. Figure 4.1 (on page 38) shows the most basic and obvious possibility for the very first slow penetration. A thick flat pillow can be placed under the buttocks of the woman in order to raise the level of the pelvis and bring the vagina closer to the penis. The raised pelvic position will also change the angle of the vagina slightly, which enhances and deepens the connection between the penis and the vagina.

Eye contact is easily managed here and will have a strong impact on the experience of gradual penetration. Lovers can allow their eyes

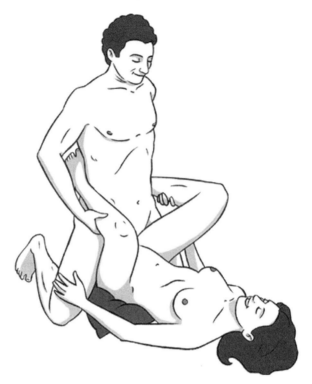

Fig. 4.1. Middle position, man kneeling
(with pillow to raise woman's pelvis)

to meet in a soft, inviting way as described in the exercise at the end of chapter 3. Eye contact can be held for the duration, although partners may close their eyes any time they wish to feel more attuned to the interior of their own bodies. One partner can have eyes open, the other closed—choose whatever brings more awareness into the situation. Do note that with closed eyes it is possible to drift away a little, and become slightly absent. It's also easier to get lost in sexual fantasy when your eyes are closed.

After a time, when the man has entered the woman fully, he can at any time change position, as illustrated in figures 4.2 and 4.3. In slow and gradual steps the man can eventually come to rest gently lying on top of his woman. In this position eye contact is often possible, other times not. It really depends on how you lie and the relative position of the two pairs of eyes.

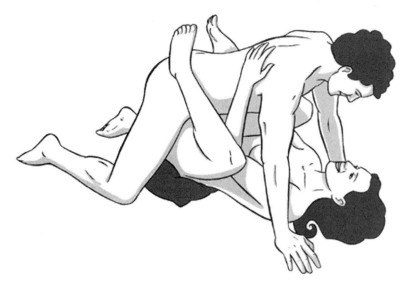

Fig. 4.2. Middle position, man on hands and knees
(with pillow to raise woman's pelvis)

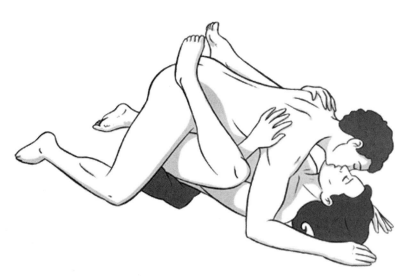

Fig. 4.3. Middle position, man lying forward, half kneeling
(with pillow to raise woman's pelvis)

Figure 4.4 shows another position option for extended slow penetration, in which both man and woman are lying on their sides. The man is actually lying between the woman's legs. In this position it is easy to make a slow, conscious journey and at the same time hold eye contact.

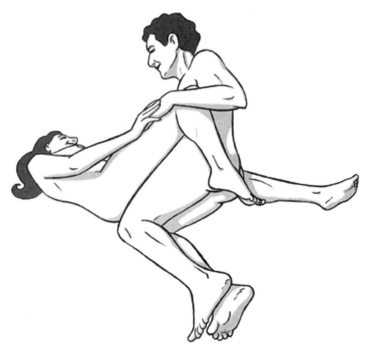

Fig. 4.4. Couple rolled to one side

Pain or Burning Sensations

It may be that the woman experiences some pain, even at the very entrance or perhaps just an inch inside the vagina. If a woman experiences any slight (or severe) sensation of burning or stinging in the tissues of the vagina as the man travels slowly inside her, she should communicate what is happening and ask him to stop in that uncomfortable place for several seconds. It is strongly advised that when he stops, the man also then pulls back a fraction so that the burning sensation or tension is reduced. This fraction of space allows tensions to move. In any case, stay with the penis head wherever pain presents itself.

Many men report that when they are slow and sensitive they can feel exactly what is happening within the vagina. The head of the penis is able to sense when and where the vaginal tissues are tight, hard, soft, receptive, defensive, relaxing, or melting. (This aspect will be addressed in depth in chapter 8.) It may take some time until the vaginal tissues relax sufficiently to allow the man to continue the entry. The time it takes is the time is takes. There is no hurry and no place for speed when it comes to entering a woman's body.

The woman can support herself by breathing deeply into her belly, taking her awareness and inner attention deep into the vaginal tissues as she relaxes and widens the canal. As she does so, the vagina becomes more receptive and welcoming, and man will immediately perceive this internal invitation, a giving way or yielding in the tissues. Buried feelings can also come to the surface for release and expression, which is a significant aspect of healing that we will address later.

STILLNESS AS AN ASPECT OF SLOWNESS

Slowness includes stillness. Slowness can transform into stillness and nonmovement at any point in which discomfort is experienced, when the "end" of the canal is reached, or when the man has arrived as far as he can go. There should be no pushing into or pressure on the cervix, which is the very sensitive entrance to the womb. Pressure can be very painful for a woman, so man must take care to pull back a fraction of an inch until pain is not experienced so that woman is able to relax and be open and receptive to the penis.

Moments or minutes of stillness can be extended to hours, if that is what both people wish. Space allows for the interplay of dynamic and receptive forces, and time allows them to respond to each other more fully. Sustain and stay with the stillness of the penetration before resuming movement. Man can hold (or intentionally direct) his awareness into the root or base of the penis and also into the head, which is like a highly sensitive and powerful magnet (see chapter 8 on healing).

To support his dynamic qualities man can imagine light energy, or gold, or love emanating from the root of his penis. While you are paused, consciously take a breath into the belly. Then scan the body by relaxing the shoulders, jaw, belly, genitals, and so on. Scan the body from head to toe and release tensions, because these cause a contraction in your energy field. Conscious relaxation of any body part will usually trigger a delicious deep breath as a wave of fine cellular sensation courses through your body in celebration. Enjoy and value being in the sexual experience without having the feeling that you have to do something. Enjoy simply being. All that is needed in the sense of doing or effort is to inwardly direct the attention to the body, and particularly into the genital tissues. Direct your awareness not only to the external surface and head of the penis but also into the very cells that comprise the tissues and muscles of the penis. For woman, move your attention from the clitoris into the tissues and muscles of the vaginal canal.

Pause for a little bit to enjoy the "now" before moving on, and then, when you sense it's the right or fitting moment, continue onward or move very slowly in the opposite direction. Halt every so often and feel into the experience; feel what you feel. Give the genitals space to become alive to themselves and alive to each other through your inner attention. Remember again the maxim, "Where attention goes, energy flows." The genitals are now "in a position" that makes inner sense to them, and the experience of new dimensions can become a reality.

Slow movements can be repeated over and over again, although you will discover that each move feels unique. What you feel and how you feel changes on each and every occasion. The bottom line is that we are wanting to establish a "correspondence" of genitals, and we put them in a position to behave according to the inherent polarities of receptive and dynamic. In normal sex the correspondence of these opposite forces is usually not happening. When we use the genitals in a mechanical, rubbing, friction-type way it certainly causes quite a stir, but at the same time it blocks access to the subtle inner potential. Through fast movement the genitals get overheated and overcharged, finally finishing up in orgasm. Being slow and still, however, allows a gently flowing cool stream of vitality to arise between them.

It is empowering to experience these subtle yet vital forces in the body, because individuals begin to feel more secure and authentic. Man feels and looks more man-like, more masculine; while woman feels and looks more womanly, more feminine. Both look younger, radiant, and relaxed. Having such experiences makes a qualitative difference to our lives with the feeling that we are stepping into a new relationship altogether.

ROTATING POSITIONS AROUND THE GENITAL CONNECTION

From time to time you will need or wish to move your bodies around to find new positions, and again relax into them. A part of the body, say the legs or back, will get uncomfortable after a bit, and when this happens, it's an appropriate time to move on. A change of position can be done at any time, after five, fifteen, or fifty minutes, whatever is required. It will bring fresh energy into the situation; you will experience yourself as more alive, alert, and sensitive. One of you will communicate your wish to move, and then you can move in unison according to the rotating style illustrated in figures 4.5 and 4.6 on pages 44–47.

Physical discomfort can be a major distraction. Instead of tuning in to the pleasure of sensitivity, your awareness is dominated by pain or discomfort. Or sometimes you may feel sleepy, a bit uninvolved, or a bit absent. A shift in position is a good remedy in these kinds of situations.

Whenever you move together the penis stays in the vagina, and you both move around with this connection as the focal point. You do not disconnect. If the penis happens to slip out, simply slip it in again. The intention behind rotating positions is to maximize the correspondence of the penis and the vagina, to keep them connected while changing position, and to bring more variety and quality into the exchange.

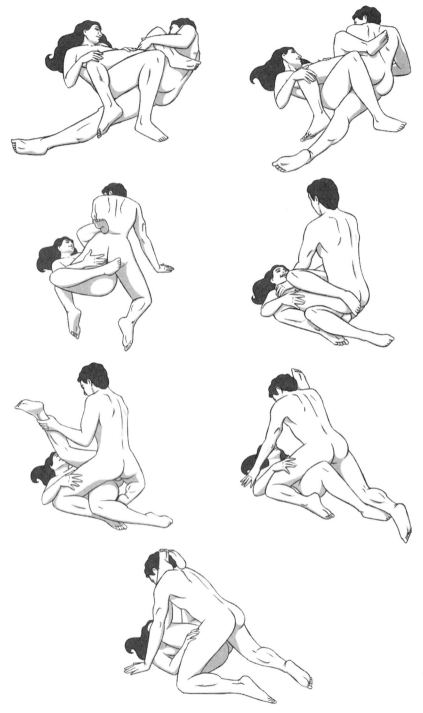

Fig. 4.5. Sequence of rotating positions through front

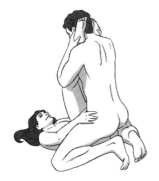

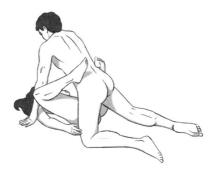

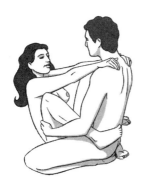

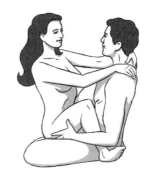

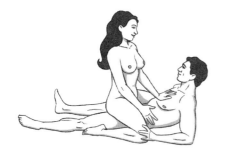

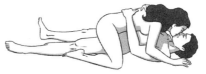

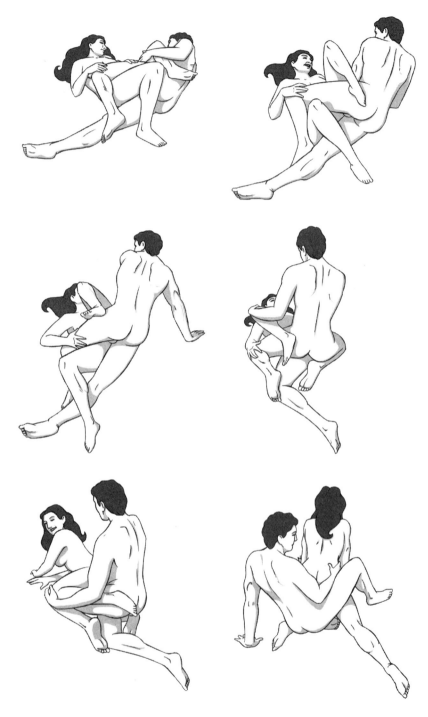

Fig. 4.6. Sequence of rotating positions through rear

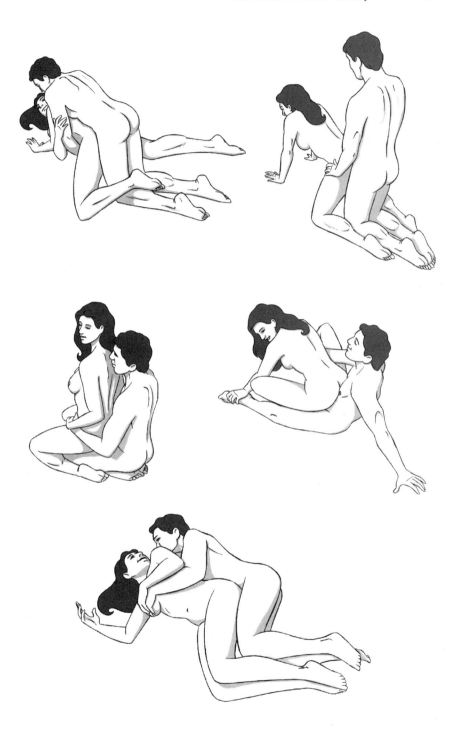

SOFT PENETRATION, ENTRY WITHOUT ERECTION

At times, especially when there is an intention to keep the temperature cooler through reducing excitement, it is not unusual to have no erection. In the usual approach, having sex is not an option without an erection—when erection fails, sex fails. However, in slow sex union is always an option because putting the penis in while soft and relaxed has great value, is easy to do, and comes highly recommended. A soft start to sex can become a regular thing, and you may find yourself choosing it as the optimal way to proceed with slow sex. A slow soft approach takes the pressure out of the situation because you can unite at any time you choose. Union is not dependent on stimulation, excitement, or erection.

Figure 4.7 illustrates the easiest position for penetration when there is no erection. Man lies on his side while woman lies on her back, and their legs intertwine in scissors-like fashion. It is recommended that this position be explored from both sides, with man lying first on one side of his body and then on the other. One side is likely to feel more familiar, cozy, and comfortable for you. The other side may feel more challenging in the sense that more is demanded of you in terms of awareness.

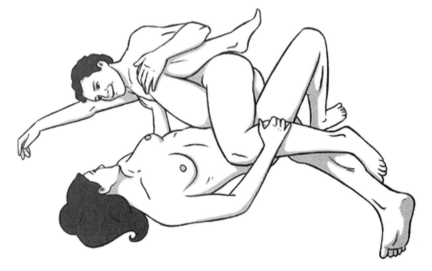

Fig. 4.7. Scissors position for soft penetration

This side-scissors position is only a suggestion for an easy starting point. The position per se is of no great significance, except that it is a very relaxing position in that both are lying down and no one is on top. It's a curious thing that the person taking the position on top generally feels compelled to do something in order to justify being in that upper position. This is man's basic sexual reality because he is more frequently on top, the missionary position being very popular. But if a woman is sitting on top of a man, she will notice a similar performance pressure, an escalated need to do something. When lying on their backs or sides, both women and men do not feel such a clear, strong drive to "do." In the scissors position man is, in fact, lying on his side, which is similar to the sleeping position, and can easily remind him of sleep. When the side position is mantained for quite a while it's not unusual for a man to drop off to sleep on occasion. Women on the other hand, who are lying directly on the back, will find it less easy to fall asleep in this scissors position. A short sleep can be regenerating, so this is not a matter for concern. If the sleeping becomes a habit, though, it's good to do some exercise before getting into bed, and to change position more often.

The side position is one from which many other positions can gradually be reached, through delicately rotating around the genital connection as illustrated earlier in figures 4.5 and 4.6. Yes, it's usually possible with a soft relaxed penis, and remember, should the penis slip out it is easy to slip it in again and continue. Other suitable positions for managing soft penetration are those suggested earlier in figure 4.3, where man kneels in the middle, and figure 4.4, where the couple is rolled over to one side (see pages 39 and 40).

Woman Inserts Man's Penis in Scissors Position

Before you move into position, it is recommended that you gently lubricate your own genitals, as described earlier in this chapter, or lovingly lubricate each other's. Do whatever feels right in the moment. As soon as you are oiled up, move into the side position as shown above and bring your pelvises close together, with the vagina opposite the penis. From here the woman can proceed by taking the penis in her two hands and gently rolling back the foreskin or any tissues around the head of the penis, pulling down toward the root of the penis. The idea of this is to expose the head's magnetic surface as much as possible in order to bring increased awareness to the radiant, dynamic qualities inherent in the penis.

Then, as shown in figure 4.8 below, woman (who should have short, rounded fingernails so that she does not scratch the vagina or penis) makes a two-pronged fork with the first two fingers of both hands. Place one finger fork (try the left hand) firmly at the base of the penis and hold the fingers there to stabilize the penis. Place the forked fingers of the other hand (the right) directly on either side and behind the rim encircling the head of the penis. Squeeze the fingers together so that you have a gentle, yet firm grip on the penis. And then pull the penis toward your vagina. When the head arrives at the entrance of the vagina you can push it a little way into the vagina. Pull the fingers back a little, then take another gentle grip on the penis, and walk or feed the penis even farther into the vagina. And then repeat the walking or feeding movement until you have pushed the whole length of the penis into you. Naturally, to do the insertion in one smooth, seamless move will take practice, so at first you may manage to get only the head, or a couple of inches, inside you. This is an

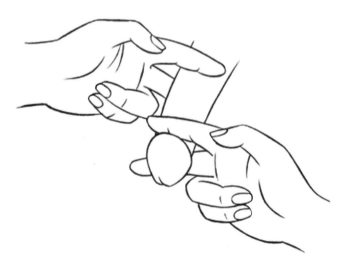

Fig. 4.8. Woman's finger position holding penis for soft insertion

excellent start and in time, when you get the knack of putting a relaxed penis into your vagina, doing so becomes second nature.

It is important to note that woman must keep her vagina relaxed and wide as she inserts the penis. Often her head is raised to look between the legs at what her hands are doing, but this move of the head tightens the abdominal muscles and the vagina. Once the fingers are in position, then woman should lie back and relax before she begins to insert the penis. When the insertion is complete and genitals are connected, wrap your legs around each other and bring your pelvises firmly together.

Bringing the bodies together in this limited-excitement way opens up all kinds of other possibilities during the sexual exchange. Just leave it up to the genitals, supported by your consciousness, and they will know how to communicate in a way that may even surprise you. It is important not to expect anything like what you have known before, and to share in words what you are feeling within. For instance, when a man hears from his partner that she can feel energy radiating from his soft relaxed penis, that is a great relief to him. Discovering that the penis has certain qualities, even if he himself cannot feel them, is very reassuring and relaxing. And instead of worrying about erection and performance, he can relax the anus and buttocks and fall back into his body and pelvis to become aware of himself from the inside out.

SPONTANEOUS ERECTION

The possibility of spontaneous erection through magnetic intelligence is built in to the genitals. The opposite forces have an effect on each other, and the penis has the capacity to wind up inside the vagina in a snakelike coiling, probing way, without any stimulation or excitement. A spontaneous erection is a by-product of the magnetic attraction and requires no effort—it happens. You can't *expect* a spontaneous erection, because it's spontaneous. It transpires when there is a constellation of invisible factors, such as when a man and woman are innocently in their bodies and merged with the inner cellular experience. Spontaneous erection is more likely when love is in the air, or where there is an element of polarization in the field, such as when man anchors his awareness in the root of the penis, the perineum, and woman connects internally with her vagina, widening and receiving.

Man will easily be able to feel the difference between spontaneous erection and intentional erection. One will feel inwardly potent and does not need movement or stimulation to maintain, while the other will feel more hollow and disconnected from the inside and is easily lost.

QUALITY IS BASED ON SLOWNESS ARISING FROM CONSCIOUSNESS

In exploring the vagina, you can again and again ask yourself a relative question: How slow is slow? It can become like a Zen koan. The answer depends on how conscious and aware you are willing to be in each and every moment. More awareness will bring more slowness. Perhaps you will be slow as a snail with one penetration taking several divine minutes, as in millimeter . . . pause . . . breath, millimeter . . . pause . . . breath. Slowness can also slow all the way down to the stillness of non-movement, nondoing. This is not a state of deadness, but an immersion within the cellular aliveness and vitality of the body, feeling and being utterly present to what is.

When sex is cultivated with respect, love, awareness, sensitivity, and slowness, the reward is elevated, beautiful experiences of ecstatic pleasure that bring joy, love, and an increased sense of well-being.

Exercise: Become Sensitive to the Quality of Your Inner Landscape

☉ Resting in Consciousness

Set aside twenty minutes for yourself and take a conscious rest. It's as simple as this: Lie down on your back, close your eyes, invert your attention, and reside within your body.

1. First, place a rolled blanket or pillow directly behind the crease of your knees, so that the legs are slightly bent and the feet/toes turned slightly inward. This support creates a softening at the knees that helps the connection to the lower body and is a great aid to deepening relaxation.

2. Then lie back and get your head, neck, and spine into one precise line. Tuck your chin slightly toward your chest so that the back of your neck lengthens. This physical alignment is crucial, because aligning yourself in this way increases the capacity to be present.

3. Lie with your hands open, palms facing up, arms lying close to your body.

4. Close your eyes, inhale a deep breath into the belly, scan and release any tense parts of your body, and then simply be present and aware in your body. You can also use the home in your body as an anchor, as was outlined in an exercise at the end of chapter 3.

Just be in your body for twenty minutes or so. It may happen that at a certain moment you sort of slip into yourself, then beyond yourself, and become taken in by your inner world into a space of timelessness. Resting in a conscious way is refreshing and rejuvenating, and turning inward gets easier with practice. This can also be used as a form of foreplay and attuning to yourself before coming together with your partner.

☉ Dynamic/Receptive Pole Variation

The preceding exercise can be slightly varied by moving the hands and placing them over the groin area, palms down on either side of the pubic bone. Then follow the steps for the aligned body position as outlined above, resting at home in your body, alive to the vitality in your cells.

After a while, man can focus his attention internally to the perineum, a knot of muscle at the root of the penis. Imagine a thread of light or warmth connecting this area to the inner home. And in the same way, woman can draw her attention into the vaginal canal, soften and widen the muscles, and rest easily with the awareness within.

5

THE SEXUAL POWER
OF RHYTHM

Rhythm is an integral part of the universe, nature, and human beings. There is rhythm in the seasons and as a pulse, in the ebb and flow of life. The very same pulse beats within each of our hearts, no matter how different our individual realities may be. We are similarly subjected to the rising and setting of the sun, and the waxing and waning of the moon. In the absence of rhythm there will be an absence of life. There are many rhythms in the human body, in addition to our basic heartbeat. Each of the visceral organs, such as small and large intestine, liver, gallbladder, stomach, and so on, has its own individual and precise rhythm and repeating pattern of movement. There are even rhythms in the brain and spinal cord, as well as three subtle levels of respiration in the body.

Perhaps the rhythm most overlooked—and therefore most neglected, even in our twenty-first century—is a rhythm truly basic to human sexual expression, the different rhythms of man and woman. In sex it is generally assumed that we have the same rhythms, that our bodies get turned on in the same way and at the same time. But this is not true. On occasion, most of us have experienced meetings or phases of being totally in tune, but as a general rule, we are different.

MAN AND WOMAN
HAVE DIFFERENT RHYTHMS

Men's and women's bodies open up, or warm up, at varying speeds. Man is fast and woman is slow as a direct result of the bodies being equal and opposite forces. The discrepancy is not psychological, despite the myth that men enjoy and want sex more than woman do.

Nature designed man and woman as complementary forces of dynamic and receptive. Dynamic is "positive" and ever ready, as most men will agree, but this is not necessarily true for women. The reason for the slowness or lack of immediate readiness on the part of woman is that the quality of receptivity is an "absorbing" force, one that can also be described as passive or "negative" polarity. A receptive force will come alive when time and space is granted for the sexual temperature to rise and equal that of man. This is a basic requirement for the full sexual metabolism to be mobilized into existence. Only then does woman become alive as a force, equal, and truly in her feminine power.

In the early stages of a relationship there is more likelihood that woman will be present with a full "yes" at the same time as her man. Everything is fresh and new, so she is naturally propelled into the moment-by-moment experience—the mysterious present. Another basic reason for this increased rapport, or woman's yes to sex, is that she is in love and her heart is alive, vibrant, and open. The heart/breast area plays a significant role in woman's general readiness for sex, as will soon be discussed.

WOMAN'S LOSS OF INTEREST IN SEX

As the initial weeks and months of wonderful sexual spontaneity in a relationship span into years, and the situation settles into a routine, it is extremely common for women to feel an increasing reluctance to get involved in sex. And as already mentioned, the avoidance of sex by a woman is usually not something coming from her mind, in the sense that resistance is something she chooses for herself, but a very physical response in which the body just closes down and loses interest. The female body begins an involuntary and gradual withdrawal from sex because the essential quality of receptivity is not honored and given space in which to thrive. The fundamental qualities of man and woman, and the opposite qualities they bring to the sexual exchange, are totally ignored in fast sex, and the reality is that as life gets busier and the novelty wears off, sex tends to get faster and be over more quickly. As a result, in the course of time a woman will find herself hardening, losing her femininity, and becoming slightly male as a by-product and kind of defense.

I know for a fact (through the personal histories of so many couples that I meet while teaching) that the majority of men would like to have sex more often than their partners would. Yet woman is unavailable to man on the "instant" basis that he has been conditioned to expect. Instant sex is the reason for the existence of the oldest profession in the world—prostitution—because it represents to man the possibility for instant sex. Sex on demand, no fuss, no foreplay. I also know for a fact that when women have slow sex, when everything is taken with ease and leisure, then women want more sex. The solution is so simple. Some of us will remember the well-known words of an old song—that a woman likes a man with a slow hand—it is true.

So the whole issue of woman's apparent lack of availability is due to a lack of understanding of rhythm and how male and female bodies open in different ways in sex. A woman is definitely capable of a superficial opening without being fully involved and alive to the experience, without participating as a fully energized and willing body. For a woman sex can, and usually far too often does, take place inside her body when she is not really involved, except as the location. For countless centuries women have yielded to the pressure of sex, gone unwillingly into sex, without particpating and sharing equally in the act. Sex starts and finishes with such speed that for a woman's female body, there is not enough time to awaken and connect with her inner receptive qualities. Embracing the female force of receptivity is fundamental to elevating the sexual exchange.

THE OPPOSITE POLE IS CARRIED
WITHIN EACH INDIVIDUAL

The secret to awakening or equalizing the sexual energy of woman, and thereby her interest in and wish for sex, does not lie in the clitoris or vagina. The route to woman's sexual source and innate vitality is via her breasts, which, on an energetic level, are very connected to the heart.

Earlier, in chapter 4, man's penis is explained as a positive, flowing, streaming force, while woman's vagina is seen as the complementary negative, receptive, absorbent force. Over and above the specific polarity we carry in our genitals, there is an even higher level to the intelligence of our human bodies—within each individual lies the equal and opposite pole. This means that in the male body there exists a female pole that is receptive, and in the female body there exists a male pole that is dynamic. Man is part woman and woman is part man, an inner design that has been proven by chromosome studies within the past hundred years. Our bodies must have always carried this astounding higher intelligence and vibration embedded in the cells of our sexual organs. Even though humanity has been following other patterns in sexual expression since the dawn of time, the creative potential of sex and its numerous benefits continue to remain alive within us as a source of vitality, inspiration, and spiritual elevation.

The body can be visualized as carrying an inner magnet with north and south poles. Or plus and minus poles, positive and negative poles, yang and yin poles . . . name them as we wish. In man the dynamic pole is the penis and his equal and opposite negative, receptive pole is the heart and chest area. In woman, as equal and opposite force to man, the receptive pole is the vagina and her dynamic pole lies in the breasts (including nipples).

Energy Is Raised from a Positive Pole

The problem with the common approach of going directly to a woman's genital area in foreplay and sex is that the vagina is a receptive pole, a passive organ, and energy cannot be raised from a negative pole; energy can only be raised from a positive pole. So for woman this means the breasts are the true source of her sexual awakening, while the clitoris and vagina are secondary. When attention (by woman herself, and also by man) is given to the breasts there will usually be (after some time) a kind of answering or response in the vagina, which is experienced as vibration or vitality, an inner awakening, together with an increasing wish to receive the penis. Awakening the positive pole in woman gives birth to the quality of receptivity in the vagina. So any inner connection a woman has to her breasts has a remarkable influence on erection, especially spontaneous erection, as described in the previous chapter.

The Role of the Clitoris Is Not Central

In my understanding and experience there is a better sequencing of events, and that is to leave the clitoris in the background until well into the lovemaking, if indeed you want to give the clitoris any direct attention at all. Again, there are no rules, but some women feel more relaxed and serene when there is no direct contact or stimulation of the clitoris; finding it preferable when pressure happens more indirectly, for example, through the position. Many women have highly satisfying sex lives without any clitoral engagement or climax-type orgasms at all. Some women find a quick peak orgasm will act as a link to the inner regions of the vagina, increasing their sensitivity. Others will feel a loss of interest. Each woman must explore the impact the clitoris has on her ultimate sensitivity and presence, and what is true for her.

The clitoris is not central to woman's higher sexual experiences. Stimulating touch of the clitoris causes sexual excitement and makes a woman full of desire. This has the effect of tightening the vagina as it gets tense with expectation. Most men have had the experience at times of entering a woman and the vagina feels hungry, demanding, or greedy, and it's an instant turn-off. The needy quality in the vagina can sometimes cause a loss of erection in man, or an immediate ejaculation. The tension of excitement and stimulation disturbs the receptive environment and throws the two equal and opposite forces out of balance.

Some men correctly observe that in their experience some women do, in fact, like, or even demand, to have hard and fast sex. Yes, this is true, some women have adopted and display man's basic attitude, but this reflects our sexual misunderstanding. Women are usually not familiar with the inner workings of their own bodies and their essential quality of receptivity. Many women have intuitions about how their bodies function, but these signals are usually discarded and the normal style of sex chosen through fear of not being loved, fear of losing a man, fear of not being sexually satisfied, or fear of being different from other women. These fears cause a lack of trust in the body, because we do not know ourselves very well. Recently I was with a group of sixty women where I asked the direct question: "Who has recognized that you have become sort of male in the way you have sex?" Every single woman in the room raised her hand. I also asked: "Who would wish for more time before being entered by man?" Again all hands were raised. The other pertinent question I asked was: "Who has observed that clitoral stimulation affects the quality of receptivity in the vagina and the impact of the penetration?" And again all the women raised their hands. The fact is, we all know the same things about our individual bodies, and yet as a group, as womankind, we continue to move forward under a collective hypnosis, repeatedly going against the truth of our bodies.

Women have yet to discover their receptive essence and the sense of arriving home to themselves that comes through honoring the body's wisdom. I have witnessed some women in my couple's groups begin in great resistance to a less active, less clitoral approach, and usually their softer, more feminine side will feel very remote because of the conditioned identification with the harder, more male side. Our personality is formed around the sexual image that we carry. The ego is, therefore, bound to fight for its rights initially, but once the experimentation gets under way, the transformation of a resistant woman is remarkably fast. Within two or three days of first having slow sex, the hardened facade begins a meltdown, the features soften and sweetly glow, and eyes shine with the light of love. And only because the vital, slow sexual rhythm and response of the female body has been acknowledged and honored. Women are, by birth and by nature, sexually slower than men and there is nothing to be done about it. It leaves us with no real choice other than to accept, respect, honor, and be grateful for the intelligence of our complementary inner designs and rhythms.

ALLOWING TIME

Respecting bodily rhythms requires granting time. Slowness in sex means allocating real time—several hours instead of just a handful of minutes. Make a date to have slow sex, and plan on at least three hours. Don't try to squeeze sex into a busy schedule, but make getting together a high priority of the day or the week.

The three-hour time proposal does not mean you have to be sexually engaged the entire time, although you may sometimes find yourselves doing so. Pauses and breaks will occur naturally. The extended time frame creates a valley of relaxation, giving birth to a slower rhythm, one where you have time to arrive in your bodies and gently flow with the experience. Start from zero and slowly warm up, instead of going from zero to a hundred in just a few minutes. With plenty of time allotted, the exchange can flow organically, with no pressure, no goals, no onward plan. There will be moments in which natural pauses occur—for adjusting position, pillows, or bedding, having a glass of water, using the bathroom, or whatever. You can stop any time for a shower or a cup of tea. And then come back to bed, connect, and give it another whirl.

Extending the Experience

Honoring sexual rhythm also implies taking it easy in the sense of extending each element of the actual sexual experience. Take the awareness and attention to the subtlest level you can manage. Any enhanced inner perception will make you more sensuous and sensitive, as if sipping and savoring each second with delight. When you enter the very moment, time and ego disappear. If you are alive to yourself at the outset and not lukewarm or detached, you get totally caught up in another dimension, fueled by an inner power. Bodies are capable of quite extraordinary and unimaginable energy events when tuned in to and trusted to flow at their own pace and in their own rhythm.

REGULARITY AND FREQUENCY

Rhythm also relates to how frequently you make love. More often is better than less often, especially when talking about quality, life-enhancing sex. Regular is better than irregular. Like many things, the more you practice with regularity and frequency, the better you get, and the more you want to practice. The more you experience the beauty of slow sex, the more you will want to partake. When good intentions and honorable wishes lose priority, complacency and laziness can quietly slide into the equation. Then, all too easily, you are out of practice, out of rhythm with yourself and your partner. In some ways the body is like a musical instrument, and if you've ever slacked off on practicing an instrument for six months or so, you know that getting back on track looks arduous and daunting; postponement and delay become the easier option. The impetus for adventure and the desire to explore the unknown are lost, as is the opportunity to be transformed in the process.

RHYTHM AS BREATH

Breath is vital to the metabolic power of sex, as it literally breathes vitality into the moment. In one sense we have no control over our breath—our bodies automatically breathe themselves. However, breath is a rhythm that we can easily influence to great advantage.

When attention is given to the breath—the very act of breathing— you are held in the present with enhanced alertness, which will further deepen and slow the rhythm of the breath. There are several ways in which the breath can be playfully explored to varying effects. You will, however, need to stay alert to the trap of the mind, which can get distracted, caught up with what's going on and with getting it right, thereby causing a certain degree of absence.

Simultaneous Breathing

In simultaneous breathing, you both breathe in at the same time and out at the same time. The breaths are deep and slow into the belly, in the direction of the genitals (use visualization if you do not feel any sensation of breath actually arriving in your genitals), and you stay as much as possible in breath synchronicity with each other. It's best to allow the breaths to be of a similar duration. You can even extend the duration for four or five counts, for instance; not aloud, of course (except at the outset, perhaps, just to mutually set the pace). If you slip out of rhythm, which can easily happen, relax for a few breaths and then slowly begin to pick up the rhythm of your partner again. Be light and easy and avoid making the breath into something stressful.

Alternating Breathing

In this type of breathing, one person breathes in as the other breathes out. Alternating breathing gets you very involved in the body and in what is happening, as it is happening. Alternating breathing can also be connected with so-called circular breathing, which uses visualization to awaken and support the electromagnetic circular flow of energy between the bodies, as in the exercise below.

Exercise: Rhythmic Circular Breathing with Visualization

↻ Circular Breathing with a Partner

In this exercise you can use visualization to accompany the breath. The excercise can be done with or without music.

1. Start with yourself, open eyes or closed eyes, and take the attention in and down, anchoring your awareness in the body.

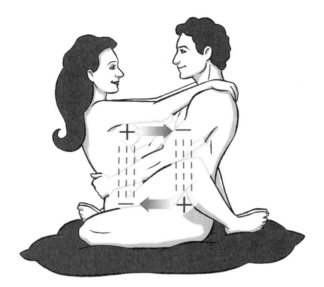

Fig. 5.1. Opposing female and male polarities
with inner magnets in alignment for circular energy flow
(in yab yum position)

2. Then bring awareness to the positive poles, man downward to the perineum (at the root of the penis) and woman upward to her breasts and especially into the nipples.

3. When you feel ready and in tune with yourself move into the yab yum position (making all suitable adjustments for comfort) and then bring your chests together (eye contact optional), and also line the nipples up so that they correspond with and directly touch each other. This can be done (and the effect felt) with or without clothing.

4. Once you are in a comfortable position, woman should imagine that light and breath is entering through her vagina on the in-breath, and flowing out of her breasts and nipples on the out-breath. She radiates light and life force into her man's chest.

5. Man can likewise imagine that he is receiving a vital force from woman on his in-breath, and in turn breathing consciously out of his perineum and penis as he radiates light, gold, and love into woman's vagina. Continue this alternate breathing and visualization for as long as you wish.

⊙ Individual Variation of Circular Breathing

By using the flame of a candle, the breathing exercise described above can also be done alone by an individual.

1. Breathe the light from the flame in through the receptive pole (the vagina for woman, the chest for man).
2. On the out-breath, return the light to the flame through the dynamic pole (the breasts for woman, the penis for man).

You can keep a circle of light flowing between you and the flame for several minutes, synchronizing the direction of your breath with the visualization of a flow or perhaps you even feel the inner cellular sensation of flowing or streaming expansion.

6

THE SEXUAL POWER
OF PLEASURE

*Opening to more pleasure can spark metabolism and
return the body to its natural state of balance. . . . What I
would like to suggest to you is that health, and by extension
any action that promotes health, is inherently a deeply
pleasurable experience.*

MARC DAVID (*THE SLOW DOWN DIET,* PAGE 110)

SENSITIVITY, THE SOURCE OF PLEASURE

Sex can be deeply pleasurable and can also benefit the health of body,
mind, and soul in many miraculous ways. Pleasure in sex is generated through giving highest priority to the rhythms of nature that
are reflected in our bodies, and giving value to, and enjoying, the
innate sensitivity that arises as a result. Sensitivity is born through
awareness, relaxation, and quality. Sensitivity and sensuality allow an
intense aliveness as a by-product of honoring the differing rhythms
of man and woman. More sensitivity creates more pleasure. With a
connection to, and awareness of, our mighty senses we find ourselves

in the optimum position to experience profound dimensions of pleasure. The pure pleasure of sex is a human birthright and one of the joys of living in a physical body.

Sensitivity indicates an awareness of, and inner connection to, the cellular aliveness inherent in the body. Sensitive does not mean ouch! this hurts or that hurts. Yes, this type of reaction is a reflection of a type of sensitivity, or in some cases a hypersensitivity, which is more related to memories in the body as a residual emotional tension or defense. However, the sensitivity required to experience pleasure at its deepest level requires an internal connection to the flesh—an awareness of the inner cosmos and all the magical sensations that can be experienced there. The key to activating the metabolic power of pleasure is to trust your body and your ability to experience pleasure.

SLOWNESS ENHANCES SENSITIVITY

The undeniable reality is that as soon as you slow down you become more sensitive. One of the remarkable things noticed by the men in our retreats is that after three or four afternoons of slow sex practice, their penises very quickly get more sensitive and perceptive. They can feel into the tissues much more deeply when their movements are slow and conscious; the penis has a much finer type of magnetic sensitivity, perception, and intelligence—different from the intense sensations experienced through stimulation. I am so often awed by the body and how quickly it responds when awareness and intelligence are brought into the sex act. Through awareness and its by-product of slowness, the tissues heal and become resensitized in a very short space of time, in both men and women. When asked, most women will admit that their vaginas are more sensitive and receptive after just a few days of making love in a more relaxed (and not focused on orgasm) way. The body regenerates as soon as it is granted the space and the trust. Pleasure loves slowness. Pleasure loves sensuality.

THE SHIFT FROM
SENSATION TO SENSITIVITY

To increase pleasure we need to increase sensitivity, slowness, and sensuality. We need to tune in to our many senses: breathing as a sense of smell, touch as a feeling sense, eyes as a receiving sense, and awareness as a witnessing sense. Sensation as we commonly understand it is not truly sensitivity. Sensation is often the response of an erogenous zone or sensitive area to some form of external stimulation, but this is not cellular sensitivity. To become more sensitive requires that we make a shift away from sensation, which is based on stimulation and excitement, involves the other (the stimulus), and includes the buildup of tension. Certainly sensitivity can also be sensational, but not in the usual sense. Sex today relies almost entirely on stimulation and sensation, which actually leads, in the long term, to less sensitivity.

It has been scientifically proven that long-term overexposure to sensation leads to an ultimate loss of sensitivity. At the end of a couples retreat several years ago, a scientist who had participated told me that the loss of sensitivity in the face of intensity of stimulation had been scientifically proven in the second half of the nineteenth century by German physiologist Ernst Weber and physicist and psychologist Gustav Fechmer. Their research, formulated as the Weber-Fechmer law, is the theory of the relationship between stimulus and experience. Their research showed that the change in intensity of a sensation varies in increments proportional to the relative change of the stimulus. Today this is known to be true for every sensory channel within its range of dynamics. A simple example would be to light a match in the darkness. In this instance the light is like an explosion, but if you do the same in bright sunlight, it is barely perceptible. More sensation correlates to less sensitivity, and less sensation correlates to more sensitivity. Instead of habitually seeking more and more sensation, you can begin working on your senses so that you become capable of feeling the subtle, yet vital life force moving through you.

Fast, hot sex desensitizes the body, and especially the penis and vagina, because it is mechanical and extroverted, dependent on sensation. The more sensation is increased, the more innate sensitivity is lost. This probably accounts for the widespread problem of impotence. Impotence represents a loss of sensitivity and awareness. A man through overstimulation slowly becomes dead to himself, and then to others, eventually unable to respond to the sensation of a strong stimulus.

Very often the fear of not feeling (in man or woman) can be the impetus for seeking sensation. At least you know for sure you can feel *something* in that particular situation. With relaxation everything is wide open, and the fear of not feeling or the fear of the unkown will keep many of us in sensation-seeking patterns. The important thing as you begin to explore is not to expect the same things as you have known up to now. You begin to experiment and gather your own body of experience. You need to become more sensitive, relaxed, and open, and thereby more capable of feeling into yourself. And you need to discover the value of the subtle. There is a shift from mind to body, from sexual desire where the focus is up and out on the periphery in extrovert style, toward the opposite—a full inversion, diving in and down into the body. Finding rest at home. The more aware, relaxed, and present you become (where true relaxation equals aliveness), the more sensitive you will become. Sensitivity creates presence, so they go hand in hand.

SLOW SEX IS COOL SEX

Slowness is always kind of cool, and yet not cold. There's a kind of distance, but not disconnection, when you are inwardly absorbed by more subtle happenings in your body, and not caught up in making sex hot and exciting. For sure, fast, hot sex can have the immediate appearance of satisfaction—and that's its curious appeal—but over time its stresses and goals can easily give you the sense of going around in circles. Eventually nothing exciting beckons on the horizon. Sexual boredom, or eventual lack of sex, is one of the main reasons why it becomes difficult for a couple to sustain a relationship over many years, and these days the frequent change and exchange of partners is considered the way to address such an unsatisfactory situation. Sexual frustration and sexual desire underlie the increasingly high demand for pornography, which is invariably focused on stimulation and sensation. When sex is equated with heat, excitement, and stimulation, it can make a man numb to himself, encapsulated by a world of sexual fantasy.

Believing that sex is based on the heat of excitement, we keep looking down the path of sensation when, in fact, we should turn in on ourselves and look at (and feel) the ecstatic sensitivity of our inner cellular vitality. But you need to cool down so that you can bring the focus back to yourself, where you are rooted in your body and your being, not focused on excietment, orgasm, or on your partner. The thing about coolness is that it is eternal, it does not burn out and come to an end the way jumping around in excitement eventually does. Being hot all the time will eventually become exhausting! A cool stance gives you some centering and repose, and at the same time will have you gently plugged into something much vaster than you. There are no rushes, rises, or falls.

Staying cool is easily done by holding your attention in your own body. Find an inner home to anchor your awareness and attention, as described earlier in the exercise at the end of chapter 3. From this sense of rooting yourself in your own body (you can also include the whole spine as your midline) comes an absorption in the enchantment of your inner cosmos. From here, from your very center, you can expand endlessly outward into the beyond.

INCREASING THE CAPACITY TO PERCEIVE THE SUBTLE

Sensitivity is pure pleasure and increasing our sensitivity makes us increasingly capable of feeling the subtle. Sensitivity requires that you give yourself the opportunity and space to perceive subtle sensations. And to identify them as a source of pleasure. You tune in to yourself on a much finer level and doing so makes the body more porous; the cells become more vibrant and fill with light. With accumulated tension over years, the body becomes tight, and eventually hardened, which makes it dense, less porous, less sensitive, and less receptive. Relaxation and the inner expansion that follows is basic to the quest for more sensitivity and pleasure. Relaxation implies turning inward and getting closer to yourself, first and foremost, on an inner level. And it is this closeness to yourself, your own inner friendliness and familiarity, that will bring you the experience of greater closeness and intimacy with another person. The other doesn't change; *you* change. And because you transform your own approach, your partner usually follows suit and responds with sensitivity and presence.

It's an incredible and mysterious alchemy. The pleasure and delight of nature's genital intelligence and sensitivity is something that will usually grow with time and exposure, meaning that you actually make love and open up to experience deep fulfilling pleasure. Not a pleasure that leaves you wanting it again and again, but a pleasure that nourishes, fulfills, and uplifts you. When you are turned on by sex, when you experience sex in full-bodied pleasure, there is an impact on the entire sexual metabolism. A fast sexual style and fast lifestyle close a doorway of perception that decreases your pleasure threshold. There is a fascinating mind-body-spirit connection linking sexual metabolism, pleasure, and beauty. Opening to the finer pleasures of sex presents a thrilling arena that invites love and transformation.

7

THE SEXUAL POWER
OF THOUGHT

Many years ago I heard it said that a man thinks about sex every two to three minutes, and a woman, every five to six minutes. Whatever the real statistics are, there is no doubt that sexual thoughts tend to dominate our minds. Even when we don't generate the thoughts ourselves, sex-related thoughts are continually provoked through advertising, media, films, pornography, jokes, and fashion. It is safe to say that the majority of us think about sex more than we actually have it.

The sexual domain is powerfully influenced by pleasant, painful, fantasizing, guilty, lustful, desirous, angry, disrespectful, disappointing, frustrating, or insecure thoughts. For many, the associations with sex are neither positive nor pleasant, and sex tends to be blanketed by a mantle of disappointment and discontent. In some individuals, searching for satisfaction can reach the level of an obsession or addiction in an attempt to fulfill seemingly endless and unfulfillable urges.

People think about sex more often than they engage in it because humans are not really having enough sex of the fulfilling and sustainable variety. As a result, our sexual energy is repressed and becomes diverted, sometimes in unhealthy, unloving ways.

THOUGHT AS DISTRACTION

The problem with our thoughts is that they are an aspect of the mind, separate and distinct from the body, where sex physically takes place. However, thoughts can have a strong impact on the body and alter the ensuing experience. Thought basically disconnects us from the inner subtle experiences of the body. I noticed how easily I slipped into irrelevant thoughts right from my first sexual experiences. I remember being shocked to notice myself having arbitrary thoughts during sex, thoughts that were not necessarily sex related. Any old thing would pop up and disturb my involvement in the present. In my innocent virginal imagination, sex should have been an all-consuming, overwhelming event that would somehow take control of me and obliterate my thoughts. But instead, when I found myself "still thinking," I remember being quietly devastated.

The propensity of the mind to drift off into thought and away from the body is something I have continued to observe, both in daily life and during my exploration of sex. It's like a lateral shift. The mind slides in sideways, distracts, and effectively darkens the inner light and subtle sensations present in the body. However, the instant the shift to mind is detected or observed (using the awareness), the reverse shift can be managed very easily. The inner connection to the body can be reestablished and the inner sensations resumed. It is not as if the inner sensitivity actually goes away in those moments of thinking. The inner cosmos continues to spiral and swirl in spite of us, but the finer level of subtlety and sensitivity moves out of the awareness and becomes swamped by thoughts.

THOUGHT AS SEXUAL CONDITIONING

Unsatisfactory sexual experiences and unhappy associations with sex are not due to sex per se. Definitely not. Sex in and of itself is God-given and divine, and we will explore the sexual power of the sacred in chapter 8.

The negative associations of sex are more a result of the way in which sex is used by the human race. It's focused on the spilling of semen and continuation of the blood line, and this has many consequences, some visible, others less visible. The stresses of survival and the ensuing speed with which we live our lives disconnect us from the cellular vitality of the body. As humans we generally turn sex into something profane by not being able to manage our magnificent sexual force with wisdom and insight.

The subject of sex is seldom directly addressed. Regularly I ask the participants in my groups, "Who received a sex education?" Only on occasion will one or two, out of a total of fifty people, raise their hands. And when I then ask, "And was it helpful?" the raised hands are slowly lowered. Not always, but usually. At school we are taught biology and the basics, the sexual organs and process of reproduction, but nothing is said about how to actually engage oneself, express oneself, and share of oneself during the sexual act. The sex education we receive is accidental.

In truth, anatomical and biological reproductive information about sex is of no real support to us, and at the same time, sex is a vital force that nobody can really avoid. Instead, we are directly influenced and affected by the powerful sexual vibrations in the atmosphere. We hear things, we see things, we feel things, we imagine things, and so become unconsciously conditioned by these mighty, yet invisible forces. The style of sex that we know is an acquired condition, and it is not necessarily how we are born to be in sex.

This unconscious conditioning has altered our minds and our psyches, and penetrated the very cells of our bodies. The orgasm urge holds us firmly in its grip, almost as if we are under a certain spell, which is why it is virtually impossible to conceive of another style of sex. Especially as we get a bit older and more settled in our sexual ways. My observation so far has been that the young couples (ages eighteen to thirty) who come to our seminars are noticeably more open to exploring and finding new ways than couples in their forties, fifties, and sixties, who are more identified with their sexual personalities.

When we are young we are more innocent, and our bodies and

psyches are more pure. We are not encumbered by a sexual history that has accumulated over years. Younger people need only a small shift; it feels natural and easy for them to be aware and relaxed, whereas for someone older, incorporating these aspects into sex can feel like an imposition on their expression.

This situation is a by-product of our sexual conditioning and a lack of insightful sex education. We are not to blame for the limitations imposed on our sexual expression, and at the same time it is good to realize that the situation is a direct result of blindness to our true sexual design. It is as if we have been looking through glasses that restrict our vision, so we cannot see the wider or higher purpose of sex. And perhaps our sexual approach is understandable, because until a certain point in time, humans were compelled to reproduce and master their environment to ensure their survival. Their whole orientation has been to focus their attention outside of themselves. There has been neither opportunity nor encouragement to explore the inner workings of human sexuality. And most of those who have turned away from the material outer world to the inner world have been religious groups promoting withdrawal from the body and denial/repression of the relentless urges of the flesh. Sexual energy cannot be tamed or contained, so it has been forced underground to become something secretive, impure, and guilt ridden.

When sex became a sin it was swept under the rug and reappeared again as secretive short-lived sex and thoughts circling around in our heads. The thoughts persist because of the relative lack of sex. When you don't have satisfying sex you fantasize or dream about it, you pervert it, or you masturbate. When we have eaten a fully satisfying meal we stop thinking about food. When we are hungry we look at the object of our desire in a very different way from when we are satiated.

THOUGHT AS DESIRE FOR ORGASM

Orgasm as the goal of sex is a reflection of our sexual conditioning. Some men and women who have explored sex in depth have shared their observation that the thought of orgasm is needed before there is the desire for orgasm. In other words, the goal is basically a mindset, and the body can be talked into it. I have observed this as well. Thought precedes compulsion, desire, and orgasm, and the exciting-climax fixation is, in fact, part of our inherited conditioning in sex and becomes a great disturbance in true human sexual expression.

THOUGHT AS SEXUAL FANTASY

For many people sexual fantasy goes hand in hand with sex. Fantasy can fuel sex. It turns you on, sets you on fire, and keeps you burning, especially when the actual reality fails to do so. It is considered totally acceptable to use sexual fantasy as a stimulant, and even encouraged as a way to find sexual satisfaction. Fantasy has become the trigger for the physical responses of the body, but fantasies are a projected world and not happening for real, so therefore have absolutely nothing to do with the inner reality of the human body. In fact, fantasy makes us absent to the present. The function of pornography, which is a type of fantasy, is to stimulate the imagination and inflame the body. Regular use can cause a dependence on sexual stimulation and excitement, and slowly the body's true sensitivity will be lost and become unresponsive, going kind of numb through overuse and misuse. Impotence is a sign of the body losing its innate sensitivity to the pressure and tension of stimulating sex.

Eyes open or maintaining receptive eye contact is the best way to reduce sexual fantasy. Eyes open anchors you in the present, in your immediate situation, and helps you to avoid drifting off into a world of fantasy.

POSITIVE THOUGHT AS VISUALIZATION OR IMAGINATION

Thoughts directed in a positive way can anchor the mind in the actual bodily reality and counteract the "absence" of fantasy or distracting thoughts. Our minds have a tremendous influence over the body and its responses, often to our detriment, but fortunately also very much for our benefit. When there is a change in mind about sex, followed by a new kind of experience, there will be a corresponding change in the nature and content of the thoughts one has in relation to sex.

The power of thought in the form of visualization or imagination (as opposed to fantasy) can be used with intention to connect with the inner realms of the body. This is a world apart from sexual fantasy and stimulation. Visualization or the imagination can help to cultivate "right thoughts" in relation to the body, so that its inner wisdom can be awakened and expressed. You imagine and support what is—something that *does* exist, and not something that does *not* exist, as is typical of fantasy. Imagination awakens energy or energy follows the imagination, and soon these extraordinarily delightful subtle inner sensations actually will begin to be felt.

A few examples of how visualization can be used: Visualize light vibrating in your cells, the color gold streaming and flowing through your body, or connecting your own positive and receptive poles. Or man can visualize energy, love, light, or gold flowing from his penis as a positive pole. And woman can imagine receiving these golden light emanations into her vagina. Woman can use her imagination in the same way and visualize love energy radiating from breasts and nipples, where her positive poles lie. Man can imagine the love and light being received into his heart and chest.

RIGHT THOUGHT AS INTENTION

Making a change to our sexual patterns usually does not happen accidentally; it requires intention and commitment. Any intention and commitment should not become a tension; it's more a matter of the willingness to pay attention. It's a relaxed orientation that includes intentionally using the awareness in order to make a shift from being mechanical and routine to being conscious and spontaneous—to going with the flow. The attention is being "inverted" and shifted back to the intelligence of the body. To help support any intention, a willing spirit, curiosity, and a sense of adventure are definite assets when stepping into the unknown.

Some kind of intention is needed because what we are attempting to do by breaking sexual patterns runs counter to centuries of collective beliefs and experience, so there is very little available in the way of external support. With the new understanding that the intelligence already lies within your body, that the secret lies inside you, there will be a slow evolution of experience that brings many benefits and blessings, and these will support a corresponding gradual shift away from fixed sexual habits.

POSITIVE THOUGHT AS REMEMBRANCE

The practice of remembrance requires awareness. Remember that first and foremost you are a body—and give it a loving thought. The body is so close it's easy to overlook its significance. It's the key, it's the bridge to the higher self. Instead the body is taken for granted and we search for a connection to the Divine outside of ourselves. Certainly the human is more than just a body, but that more follows later on as a by-product, or as a consequence of being rooted in the body, living in the awareness. At any moment during any day, fall back into your body with your awareness, scan your body, and release any tension or holding. Breathe deeply and slowly and just be suspended in the moment, as you hold the awareness within your body for several seconds. Remember, you are more than the mind; your basic truth is the body. The body is not there simply to escort and carry the mind around. The physical form is given to us to serve as a bridge to divine realms. Through intention and with awareness, humans naturally move on to higher spiritual dimensions.

The inner remembrance of any previous ecstatic experience (it is recorded as light in your cells) can be used as a very powerful means for continuing inner transformation and deepening sexual practice.

8

THE SEXUAL POWER
OF THE SACRED

S ex has long been associated with the spiritual and the sacred, in the East as well as in the West, as mentioned in the introduction. Statues and paintings in thousands of ancient temples and places of worship reflect the spiritual orientation of earlier cultures. Sex in its sacred phase is transformed into a generative, creative spiritual force, which is a higher expression than its reproductive aspect. Sacred sex is focused on generating more vitality and life for oneself and maturing as an individual, rather than using sex to produce another life. Sex becomes sacred when you honor the intelligence of the body and create the situation and space for the Divine to enter. To receive the Divine you will need infinite nothingness inside you, because you are inviting the whole of existence into you.

ENGAGING THE
METABOLIC POWER OF THE SACRED

Slow, sensual sex is a direct passage into the gentle and sacred arms of the Divine. The miracle is that each and every person who wishes to is able to gain access to the sacred. Sex is made sacred through intention and honoring the God-given wisdom of the body. We simply have to create the right environment and incorporate the universal metabolic enhancers, such as awareness, relaxation, rhythm, pleasure, and so on.

Marc David writes:

> Sacred metabolism is the chemistry ignited in the body when we are infused by the Divine. Because the Divine is the source of power behind all powers, the chemistry created when we experience the Divine supercedes all known laws of the body. Sacred chemistry is a meta-chemistry. Its effects can include or incorporate familiar psychophysiologic states, such as the relaxation response, brain-hemispheric synchronization, pleasure chemistry, immune-system mobilization, and others. (*The Slow Down Diet,* page 159)

ECSTASY IS BEYOND PLEASURE

Our innate bodily sensitivity opens the door to the Divine, easily, gently, and organically. We are designed by nature for a natural biological ecstasy, a dimension that can be described as being light-years beyond pleasure. Ecstasy is pure bliss, a sacred state of utter contentment, peace, and harmony in which the being merges with the whole of existence and falls into harmony with all that is.

The essential components of blissfulness or ecstasy are timelessness, egolessness, and naturalness. Ecstasy and bliss exist beyond the ego and the "I" that normally wants or needs something from sex. Without the "I" there is no need for orgasm and the body can drop back into the here and now. The energy is contained by remaining present to each moment. There is no moving forward, no pushing through to a climax and release in orgasm, so the vitality remains in the body.

Avoiding a climax applies equally to man and woman. However, with woman there is one difference. When a woman is able to have an orgasm easily and with no effort at all, while in a state of relaxation and being (and not doing), then orgasm is perfectly beautiful. But when a woman works with effort and intention to reach orgasm, first, she will be lacking in presence, absent through a focus on the goal. Second, she is likely to cause her man to ejaculate. And third, there will be a buildup and crescendo of physical tension, some of which is discharged in orgasm and some of which remains in the woman's energy system. These tensions can later give rise to a negative swing either on the physical level (such as vaginal irritations or menstrual pains) or an emotional level (feeling insecure, unloved, abandoned). Woman loses a geat deal of energy through the tension of much effort, just as man does. It is very interesting for a couple to begin to observe themselves hours and days after having sex, to watch their mood swings in relation to their sexual choices. When the choice is habitually excitement and orgasm, often there will be a certain level of tension between the two of you, perhaps evidenced by many emotional ups and downs that get in the way of the love you feel for each other.

When the vitality is not discharged and is allowed to gather at the base, the life force will (in time) start to rise upward. And of its own accord. This rising is not something that one can "do," as such. Actually the only thing you can really do in the situation is to stop doing the habitual orgasm thing. The situation has to be created, then the rising of energy happens by itself, as a by-product. The inner vitality is first contained, then it turns inward, a channel opens gradually, and the life force is able to spiral, or stream, or flow upward through the core of the body. When energy is contained and rises in this way, the spiritual or sacred phase of human sexual energy is stimulated into life as a generative uplifting force that nourishes the entire metabolism with life-enhancing effects.

Slow Sex Becomes a Sacred, Spiritual Practice

As sensitivity increases during sex, the exchange will become increasingly the experience of being here and now. Through remaining present and taking the awareness inward, one naturally engages with spirit and the mysterious sacred forces that breathe life into us. As many people have commented after experiencing slow sex, it feels natural and right, like a coming home to yourself.

THE INNER ROD OF MAGNETISM IS THE SOURCE OF ECSTASY

Containing the sexual energy and creating the situation for its rising involves taking a step over and beyond our inherited patterns and habits. Really what we are wanting to achieve is a shift from orgasm as a hurried event of a few seconds to the ecstasy of a timeless orgasmic state wherein the body loses sense of its physical boundaries and exists as pure, vibrant, vital energy.

The simplest route to the sacred is to take the body into consideration and honor its inner polarity. The potential for the ecstatic or orgasmic state lies within each individual because of this inner polarity, the equal and opposite poles of male and female carried within each individual, as discussed in chapter 4. Between these two opposite poles there exists a difference in potential that gives rise to an electromagnetic streaming of inner vitality, aliveness, chi, prana, or life force. There is an invisible but palpable "inner rod of magnetism" that forms a channel or passage for the flow and expansion of the subtle, electromagnetic energies that are the source of each person's orgasmic and ecstatic states.

SENSITIVITY IS THE BRIDGE TO ECSTASY

Ecstasy is not excitement. Ecstasy lies way beyond the pleasures of exciting sensations. It could rather be described as a state of pure pleasure, pure delight, and pure bliss. Through being intensely conscious and rooted in the sensitivity of the physical body, you can dissolve into a state of ecstatic bodilessness. I have found that the words from a well-known song, "you gotta get in to get out," reflect the truth. You need to merge first and foremost with your own body in order to travel and expand beyond your physical boundaries. You are born with a built-in mechanism for a natural biological ecstasy and you need to know how to harness its sacred qualities in order to move beyond the ego, time, and the physical body—to exist as pure vibrant energy.

Ecstasy Is a By-product of Coolness

Ecstasy is a cool experience. It is a state of intense inner vitality, and at the same time it is a cool and serene state. Ecstasy is definitely not hot and not at all overwhelming. Heat can and will eventually lead to some kind of a discharge of energy, whereas in coolness there is automatic retention of energy. Coolness results in an implosion, not a heated explosion. Coolness is oriented around relaxation instead of building up tension. All the contributing movements and actions are more conscious and much slower, and at times there can be stillness, too.

To invite new dimensions requires a shift of position; when you change your position you change your experience. The position can be physical, mental, or both—the two are strongly intertwined. Our conditioning is such that the body follows the mind more easily than the mind follows the body. So it's easiest to start with the mind and change our basic ideas around sex, to change our orientation to one in which the body is honored. A good physical position will have awareness at its base; the most important thing is that you have the capacity to observe yourself as opposed to being identified with a certain pattern or position. To shift your point of view on sex you need to have the capacity to step into the sexual unknown, which means finding the courage to drop the ideas you have held on to in sex, to question the identification you have with a certain style of sex. Letting go, relaxing, being present to whatever is, will pave the way to sacred dimensions.

DEFEMINIZING EXTERNALIZATION
OF THE GENITALS

Slow sacred sex is a spiritual experience because it's an inner experience. Any turn inward, away from the outer world, is a feminine movement.

Outward moving is male, inward moving is female. Our culture has conditioned us to be more outward and extroverted in so many ways, including sex, that both woman and man have lost access to their true receptive feminine qualities. This loss of the feminine is increasingly represented by what I see as an externalization of the genitals in epidemic proportions, one that is oriented on stimulation and sensation—the almost compulsory fashion of removing all the soft, silky, sensitive pubic hairs that form a glistening halo embracing the male and female genitals.

Pubic hairs are designed to protect sensitive tissues, and their complete absence represents a dramatic loss in sensitivity. Each single hair acts like a portal to the inner world of sensation because it is connected to sensory nerve pathways via its root. When hair is lightly played with or softly stroked, or even better, when the hairs are pulled gently one by one with the fingertips, there is a subtle, yet thrilling, internal sensory response. A very little can go quite a long way. Constant low-level friction with no hair to act as a buffer between the genitals may also literally desensitize (callous, if you will) external nerve endings.

This popular trend of hair removal is a very strange and distorted perception that reflects the prevailing sexual confusion. Hairlessness appears to be an attempt by adults to imitate sexual immaturity in order to send out sexual signals, which somehow depreciates adults and their behavior. A woman without her stabilizing, balancing, integrating triangle of Venus is not a mature woman. How can she be? Instead, the inviting, compelling, and appealing triangle that symbolizes the female in all her glory is trimmed into a minimal rectangle, standing almost military in beefeater style. Or often the triangle is erased completely to reveal a childlike provocative slit, with the sensitive, tender inner lips open and delicate tendrils exposed.

Exposing and externalizing the genitals through interference with pubic hair is a visible sign of a lack of self-knowledge and evidence of a sexuality that has not embraced the inner feminine. And this is equally true for both men and women. A penis that is not nestled in a glistening halo of frothy pubic hair looks unbalanced, exposed, and vulnerable. The general idea, of course, is to make the penis look larger and more impressive; however, these forms of externalization ultimately displace awareness away from the biomagnetic source of our sexual vitality.

The fashion of piercing different parts of the body, such as the testicles, penis, clitoris, navel, tongue, and nipples, also reveals an extroverted sexuality. It is another way of looking to the periphery for stimulation and sensation rather than toward the center of our innate sensitivity and the source of the feminine receptive aspect.

Wise people observe that the real reason why the world is filled with so much chaos and fear is that the primordial forces of male and female are drastically out of balance. The way to heal this radical imbalance and return to harmony is to honor and respect the powerful receptive female force for what it is, giving woman her place alongside man, and encouraging man to honor his own female side, which is inward, receptive, and embracing. Male and female cannot exist without each other—we are conceived together as one. However, the female aspect of humankind in almost all cultures in the world has suffered a loss (and abuse) of the feminine. The graceful, intuitive, loving, flowing, sweet compassionate qualities are ignored and become masked by distortions.

The imbalance between man and woman is very clearly seen in conventional sexuality, and a new understanding and vision of sex would initiate tremendous healing and balancing. I would even go so far as to say that any vision for a harmonizing shift between male and female forces would have to include at its very root a more enlightened form of human sexual contact, one that turns away from the periphery toward the center and tunes in to the design of the inner body.

THE SACRED
BALANCES AND HEALS

One significant aspect of sacred sex is the profound healing that is possible for mind, body, and spirit in ways we can't even imagine.

Reciprocal Cycle of Purification

Accumulated tension, fear, memories, and wounds from our individual sexual history are stored in the cells and can be liberated and purified from the system during slow conscious sex. As the body becomes more flexible and porous, man gradually encompasses his more positive, dynamic essence of male, and woman encompasses her more receptive and absorbing essence of female. A reciprocal cycle of purification exists between penis and vagina as a result of the interaction of dynamic and receptive forces. This means that a conscious penis will purify the vagina, and in so doing, the penis itself slowly becomes purified—more flexible, sensitive, radiant, and beautiful.

The Head of the Penis Is a Powerful Catalyst

The head of the penis is very similar to a highly sensitive magnet and when present (supported by man's consciousness) in the vagina, it acts as a powerful catalyst. It has the innate power to displace old memories, feelings, or tensions that are obstructing full receptivity. Cleansing of the poles makes the vagina more relaxed, receptive, and able to perceive the subtle. Similar tensions will also be displaced from the penis, increasing its ability to be a sensitive snakelike channel for dynamic energy.

Purification through Deep Sustained Penetration

A woman is most receptive and feminine in the deepest regions of the vagina, especially around the cervix—the entrance to the uterus. I like to refer to this place as the "Garden of Love." When woman is touched here her heart is also touched and great love arises in her body.

Purification happens with or without an erection, so a soft penis definitely has potency, but if a man wishes to travel deeper into the vagina, into the Garden of Love, he needs to have a half erection to a full erection. This can be achieved by just a little movement and avoiding getting into excitement. There should be just enough arousal for a soft, supple erection. Or an erection may arise spontaneously within the vagina, as mentioned in chapter 4.

After lubricating the penis and the vaginal entrance, woman can hold her labia open as man places the head of his penis at the entrance, waits a few moments, and then enters her slowly, stopping after a half inch or so, waiting for a few breath cycles, continuing in a little more, waiting, breathing, with man continually being present in and to his penis. Continue penetration as deep as the penis is able to manage, or until the man feels some resistance against the head of the penis. Usually a man will be touching the entrance to the uterus (the cervix) or the walls and upper boundaries of the vagina. In this area, the Garden of Love, woman is most capable of experiencing divine ecstatic energies through contact (and thereby man too). Do not use hard pressure against the vaginal tissues; this is important—pressure can compress the tissues, causing them to become defensive and closed. Once the man feels he has reached his depth, he must pull back a fraction—a hairsbreadth—so as to take pressure off the vagina and create a more porous and airy contact between the magnetic penis head and cervix. This fraction of space will enable an exchange between the male and female poles, the dynamic and receptive forces.

If a woman feels pain *at any point* during the journey of the penis deeper into the vagina, she must communicate this fact immediately and ask her man to stop and to stay exactly on that place where pain is experienced. The contact needs to be porous, so man must always pull back. Pain is a doorway in the sense that pain often reflects old memories or tensions that are held in the tissues. Hold the penis in this area for several minutes and see what wants to happen—there may be throbbing, pulsating, or electrical feelings. If any sadness or other buried feelings rise to the surface, they should be given space and expression, and honored as part of the purification process. It is not necessary to understand the source of the feelings, why and when, just allow them to pass through you. Feelings that surface should really *not* be repressed and reswallowed. By allowing old and unexpressed feelings to flow out of you, if and when they arise, there is a profound cleansing and purification on a cellular level. Over a period of time a man should explore and visit all angles and corners of the vagina, which will gradually soften, heal, and become more receptive.

Man may also experience pain, in the testicles, groin, or penis. It is very healing for a man to allow tears of sadness, insecurity, and vulnerability or whatever comes up, and gradually his penis will grow to be more sensitive, perceptive, and supple.

Positions suitable for deep sustained penetration are shown in chapter 4 in relation to man making a slow, conscious initial penetration. (See figures 4.1 to 4.4 on pages 38–40.)

SACRED SLOW SEX SUSTAINS AND STABILIZES RELATIONSHIPS

When we relax away from doing and into our being, we get in contact with the source of love—our essence—lying within ourselves. An endless source of love resides within each person. We are born in love and love is alive as light and pleasurable sensations in each cell of the body. Anywhere you feel good in your body is a place where love lives inside you. Relaxation into the being implies an awareness of, and involvement in, the body, because the body is the bridge. Awareness easily opens the way to transformation, a sacred alchemy in that awareness itself creates love. Slow sex is, therefore, by its very nature (conscious and aware) very loving sex. The awareness brought into the sexual exchange can transform the commonly repetitive act into a sacred act of love. You begin to love and respect yourself more, and this radiates to include your partner (and others), embracing them with more love, respect, and acceptance.

In the many years that my partner and I have been teaching slow sex to couples, we have been astounded to see what a powerful healing and balancing force it is and how quickly it seems to work. Sometimes couples on the brink of divorce or separation come to our retreats as a last resort to see if we have anything to offer that will help them stay together. All that we have to offer is, in fact, awareness. And this awareness is based on a new understanding of the human sexual system and how male and female are designed to unite.

We also create space daily for individual couples to have sex in privacy (always), so that they can put theory into practice. We don't need to hear from the couples how they are responding to a slow style of sex (some couples wish to share, but not all) because we can see its regenerating effects within two or three days. It's as if a breeze of light and love enters the room. The eyes shine and the faces are relaxed and radiant. The couples feel connected, while at the same time there is a unity lying within each individual. There is a simple undemanding presence and intimacy as each person settles into his or her own body. Through this awareness, self-love increases and naturally overflows onto the other. We do know as a fact that many couples remain together after being with us for this week of exploration, because they write to us afterward to say how important and life changing this education has been. Naturally the success rate is not 100 percent, but high enough to be impressive, and therefore, worthy of note. Our approach is not foolproof; rather it depends on individual awareness, curiosity, and an interest in change. Slow sex can be talked about endlessly, but it has to be tried out—put into practice so that it becomes your own experience and you feel its benefits and healing effect directly and personally.

Over the years we have witnessed a steady trickle of people returning to our retreats with a new lover. Actions are said to speak louder than words, and the return of so many, particularly men, is their living endorsement of the immense value of changing the way one makes love. Once a man has been fortunate enough to have a taste of his male potency flowing into and through a woman and being received by her, he naturally hopes to create similar experiences for himself in the future.

Basically slow sex makes sense for any couple that wishes to stay together and continue to have sex in the years after the honeymoon high fades, especially as they begin to mature and age. Classically, sex is often the reason for a separation, whereas slow sex creates a bond and a union that is beyond the need for excitement and change. It's like a ripening process in which the flavors become more refined and dimensional. And even if you separate for any reason, the experience you have had together, the learning and reorientation you have made, will stay with you and give you a good foundation for the next time you enter a love affair.

INNER SEX AS
THE MOST EVOLVED FORM OF SEX

The human body is designed so that each individual is fully able to have "inner sex" and circulate magnetic vitality. Inner sex is the highest and most evolved form of sexual expression, in that it returns to individual completion and fulfillment and is beyond, but not against, sexual union. Each of us has the capacity to circulate vitality or energy between the male and female poles in our own bodies *using the power of the awareness*. Inner sex is not self-touching or self-stimulation or masturbation. Conscious touch can certainly be used as a way to increase awareness in the positive, life-giving pole. In woman by cupping and holding the breasts, and in man, by laying the hands on the groin area or lovingly holding the penis and testicles while placing attention on the perineum. Attention on the positive pole will eventually and in time awaken the opposite pole and both will become vibrant with life. There will also be a streaming of vitality between them. And, in theory, when sensitive to ourselves, we all have the capacity to access the source of the orgasmic state lying within because we are all of similar electromagnetic design.

Many highly sensitive individuals have been blessed with the experience of the orgasmic blissful state in aloneness; for example, while out in nature or enraptured by music or dance. They are suddenly touched and graced by the Divine because of such an intense (but not tense) immersion in the body through the senses that they dissolve into the present moment. When at one with our senses there is an openness, an invitation and receptivity to the encompassing sacred forces of Divine creation.

When we have a regular long-term partner we have an opportunity to make love with another person frequently. This is the way we can help each other to access our inner orgasmic potential. We engage the inbuilt resources of the body (represented by dynamic/receptive forces) to assist ourselves in rising a few rungs on the inner ladder of growth. One thing to note is that one partner having an orgasmic experience does not guarantee that the other partner will move into the same ecstatic space or share the same experience. It may happen, but not necessarily.

Remember that the source of the orgasmic state lies within each individual and is not really dependent on another person. In a couple constellation one partner may, in fact, be more sensitive on a cellular level than the other partner, which can lead to a discrepancy of experience while having sex. For example, after some hours of making love, one partner may be entering an orgasmic state while the other is partially alseep or generally absent. The initial contact of the vagina and penis, and the ensuing inner electromagnetic circulation, initiates the process and acts as a trigger; however, the ultimate elevated experience will often be that of one person only.

Marc David writes that, "What we oftentimes label as anomalous or miraculous are simply latent biological traits activated once we are touched by the hand of the Divine" (*The Slow Down Diet,* page 160). He believes that we are at the frontier of what we know about the capabilities of the human form, and that what we know is but the tiniest fraction of what is possible. Is it possible that the fulfillment of your metabolic destiny is to be found inside you, intelligently seeded there and awaiting your discovery?

As I see it, the missing link for humans, the seed of intelligence and ultimate source of our health and well-being, lies in how we have sex, how we use our bodies and share ourselves sexually. The metabolic powers of the sacred become engaged during slow sex because there is an honoring of the eternal wisdom lodged in the body.

Marc David writes:

> . . . the sacred has its own terms that are available to all in this time and place, and whose terms are these: love, truth, courage, commitment, compassion, forgiveness, faith, and surrender. These

eight sacred metabolizers—and no doubt there are more—are sacred because such soul qualities bring us closer to the heart of the Divine, to the intelligence that created us. By embodying them we become more like the source from whence we came, more of who we are meant to be and who we know, somewhere inside, we want to be. And I'm suggesting that when activated in our system, the eight sacred metabolizers can produce profound healings and powers, metabolic breakthroughs, and rejuvenating effects on body and spirit. (*The Slow Down Diet,* page 161)

In slow sex, where relaxation, awareness, quality, rhythm, pleasure, and right thought is incorporated into our way of having sex, we begin to find ourselves naturally aligned with the eight sacred metabolic forces of love, truth, courage, commitment, compassion, forgiveness, faith, and surrender.

Love: When we enter sex with awareness we touch the being as the source of love lying within. Love is the alchemical by-product of awareness, and ordinary mechanical or routine sex can be transformed into love through engaging awareness.

Truth: When we enter sex it is our intention to live the truth of our bodies, honor and respect their intelligence, and create a situation in which we embody and appreciate our human sexual design.

Courage: When we enter sex a certain courage is needed to be curious enough about ourselves and be willing to not know. We need courage to challenge and be creative with our habits and patterns in order to live according to a higher sexual vision.

Commitment: To make a shift in consciousness, as is required in slow sex, requires commitment to the now. Commitment is part of personal and spiritual transformation. It is not an obligation, but more a sense of seeking to find out who we really are, and to make time and space for the sexual exchange as often as possible.

Compassion: With a new approach we are able to enter sex with compassion and understanding for our bodies and for each other.

We have compassion for the crucial complementary differences between male and female systems.

Forgiveness: To enter into sex requires that sometimes we have to forgive ourselves and/or others. This will usually entail releasing, through forgiveness, certain events or acts from the past.

Faith: It takes faith to leap into the unknown and trust that such elevated experiences are available to a human being.

Surrender: To approach sex in a spiritual and sacred way requires that we surrender ourselves to the intelligence of nature by relaxing into our bodies and giving way to forces greater than ourselves.

Exercise: Using Prayer to Invite the Divine

☺ Blessing Your Union

One beautiful way to begin lovemaking is with a blessing or prayer, silent, spoken, or shared.

1. Kneel or sit opposite each other and bring your hands together in prayer position in front of your chest and heart. Begin by closing your eyes, taking a breath, and relaxing into yourself.
2. When you feel ready you can open your eyes and hold a soft eye connection with your partner for a while.
3. Speak your prayer (or say it silently), and then lean forward with lowered heads and bow to each other, letting your foreheads rest together.

When you bless and pray you invite the Divine to participate in your love creation. You attract unforeseen supportive forces into the electromagnetic field around and beyond you.

Exercise: Using Ritual to Invoke the Sacred

☺ Create an Atmosphere of Love

Ritual is a powerful way of creating an atmosphere for the sacred. Following certain steps or protocol helps you to crystallize your intention and focus your awareness with the senses tuned in to the present moment. There are many ways that a ritual can be performed and many different elements that can be included. The ritual space (the bedroom, for instance) needs to be prepared and beautified so as to invite the spirits. Spirits love beauty so if you don't know many details about creating ritual, then let pure beauty be your guide. Flowers, low lights, candles, beautiful embroidered cloths, crystals, treasured or sacred objects, fragrance, and music can all be incorporated into the ritual arrangement. Having your heart in the right place is what counts most.

☺ Focus Your Sacred Intention with an Altar

An altar can be created as a focus for your intention to invite the sacred, perhaps on a small round table or in an alcove. You might like some of the following suggestions for how to arrange your altar, or perhaps you already have some ideas of your own.

- Place crystals as the centerpiece of the altar to represent and channel a certain quality, such as love or compassion, into the atmosphere.
- Arrange three crystals at the center to honor, give gratitude to, and ask for blessings from Mother Earth (the feminine), Father Sky (the masculine), and the Great Spirit that breathes life into this union.
- Flowers or a candle can also be placed in the center of the altar.
- Set any other precious, meaningful, or high-frequency objects around the central piece in a way that is energetically or visually meaningful to you.
- Photographs and pictures can also be used to invite particular energies into your sacred space.
- A glass of fresh drinking water is nice for the spirits, too.

☺ Use Ritual to Come into Your Body in the Present Moment

A ritual will usually begin with (or along the way include) some kind of prayers or blessings, as mentioned in the previous section. You may wish to work out a specific sequence of words accompanied by certain movements that you engage in as a way of beginning every time you make love. Ritualized steps function to bring us step-by-step into the body and into the present. A part of a ritual (or the whole ritual) can also take the form of a meditation, dance, or breathing exercise. There are a variety of ways that can assist us in bringing the body, the awareness, and the senses into focus and alignment.

Select something you enjoy that is meaningful to you. Even something simple like bowing down to each other and then lying down separately and relaxing into your bodies, resting in the awareness for ten to twenty minutes, is a good preparation (as described at the end of chapter 4).

☉ Move Consciously into Physical Contact

Then stand and move very slowly and deliberately toward each other, maintaining eye contact. From here you can slowly come into an embrace, kiss if you wish, then lie down together. You can also take some time to communicate to each other what you feel in your body and your heart.

Sharing your internal now experience (like a brief weather report) will help to amplify the inner experience. The acknowledgment or the recognition of what is—what exists in the present—is rewarded by the sensations expanding delightfully through the body. Speaking aloud about inner sensations also lets each one know what the other is feeling, so no guesswork is needed. This is very relaxing and supportive. Any kind of preparation that gets you more involved and engaged with the body and its sensitivity will be a tremendous support for experiencing sex in its elevated form.

9

THE SEXUAL POWER
OF THE STORY

Each individual, regardless of who we are or where we were born, has two basic stories with sex, simply by virtue of having arrived in human bodily form. There is the personal story and the human story. The personal sex story very often contains many stories, and some of them may be not so pleasing or worthy of remembering. This is not because of sex itself, but because the how of sex is based on an absence of true bodily respect, understanding, appreciation, and insight.

THE HUMAN STORY IS A SEX STORY

On the human level, the story is that sex is the most basic expression of our bodies. It is determined by our DNA and the biological programming that is set for continuation of the species, as is true for all living species on Earth. At its most superficial level, life is focused on procreation and nourishment.

From day one we live in a human body and are all similar, not at all individual. The bodies and psychologies do get influenced in many ways by different experiences and exposures, but in our essence we are all one and the same. This similarity means we have to embrace the sexual story endowed by our Creator and lying inherent in the body.

The story of the body is our three-dimensional human story and the urgent need to follow our inner electromagnetic design, so that humans can experience an evolved style of sex. Slow sex, and that means sex that has awareness as its base, represents an evolutionary step for us. There is no need to elaborate on the sexual distress and malaise present in our culture. The evidence is all around us as we witness a massive escalation in abuse and pornography, plus a sharp rise in the rate of divorces and separations based primarily on some sexual reason: boredom (and finding someone new and exciting), lack of interest in sex (woman's body closes down when her body is entered too fast), lack of fulfillment (because energy is repeatedly discharged), and so on.

Each of us, whether we know it or not, like it or not, is in an intimate, lifelong relationship with sex. Sex is a relationship that really cannot be avoided because we are genetically programmed for it. Our bodies (with amazing speed) become sexually mature in order to reproduce the species. Fortunately, if we don't have sex we don't die, but all the same, most individuals will have an ongoing relationship with sex in some form or another, whether they want it so or not. Sexual energy can be diverted and the force of it repressed, but there are significant negative consequences to repressing nature. We cannot really choose whether or not we are sexual beings, but we are definitely in a position to choose when and how we act on it.

THE PERSONAL SEX STORY

The human story all too quickly becomes a personal story, especially with the prevailing lack of insight and information about sex. Millions of people suffer as a result of negative sexual experiences. Countless lives are traumatized as a direct result of an absence of respect for innocent human beings that leads to sexual abuse and the overstepping of personal boundaries. Abuse takes place because a sexually repressed individual is controlled by sexually demanding urges (and fantasies), desires that harm others when acted upon.

Sex can be the source of tremendous personal pain, guilt, and confusion, as well as a source of attraction and great pleasure. It is indeed, then, a blessing from the Divine that slow, sensitive sex has powerful healing and balancing effects. Deep pain and confusion exists on the collective level, too, so culturally sex continues to be shrouded in a veil of darkness and secrecy that separates us from the deeper reality (and need) of the human body. We have almost no meaningful or creative insights into the true function of sex. Tremendously high levels of frustration, suffering, distress, anger, and even rage exist as a result of "unholy" sex, even if we do not necessarily recognize the connection between these emotional consequences and sex, or the lack of it.

As far as sex goes, humans are more or less on a starvation diet. Insufficient sex, as well as the briefness of most sexual interactions, leaves us undernourished on profound metabolic levels. Our quality of life is dramatically affected and reduced to the minimum. When the sexual energy is flowing (within oneself or between two people), then creativity flourishes and love ignites and spreads. Sex "rightly" used is known to boost the immune system, stimulate creativity and intelligence, and increase happiness throughout adult life. In the current state of affairs, sex comes to a standstill and many people abandon sex when they get older.

Many people take sex to extremes of sensation and stimulation (and insensitivity to themselves) while endlessly seeking "satisfaction." Pornography and visual stimulation is at an all-time high. Exploitation of children is tragically acute and on the increase. For many, masturbation, fantasy, and virtual sex are becoming more of a reality than real-time sex. Many men need pharmaceuticals, such as Viagra, to give them potency because they have lost innate sensitivity. Most men cannot control their ejaculation and many women struggle to have a climax.

SLOW SEX,
A STEP IN HUMAN EVOLUTION

As humans we are caught, without intention but by an unconscious conditioning, in the reproductive, biological, and extroverted phase of sex—brief and hot. Is this truly all that it is meant to be for us? What is our actual potential and our deeper story with sex? Slow sex enables us to step into the generative, creative, uplifting aspect of sex in which the feminine and inner workings of the body are honored and embraced. It becomes essential to our health, well-being, and sustainability at the deepest level of reality.

Couples who have done our "Making Love" retreat often return two, three, and even more times to repeat the week-long experience so as to deepen their inner exploration. The human sexual story is an unfolding; it's not something that can be fully grasped all in one shot. You have to live sex and transform its expression step by step. What usually happens is that people will begin to change and transform themselves, through the very practice itself. The whole process of transforming the sexual energy into a spiritual sacred expression is the process of becoming a witness and observer of your experience. As you go along you will begin to understand more, see more, have insights and revelations, and one by one the pieces of the jigsaw will fall into place and you'll find yourself standing in a totally different world. All the same elements will be there, but the constellation will have changed dramatically. There will have been a revolution in the way you see your personal sexual story, realizing it has become a human story that brings you back home to yourself, and returns you to your electromagnetic place in the universe.

10

YOUR PERSONAL SLOW SEX PRACTICE

Slow sex is a journey in which today counts, and each and every day counts. It's a slow journey that can extend over many years and into old age. Or so it is happening for me, and I can definitely say that I did not plan for it to be this way. Very slowly, one thing has led to another through curiosity and practice.

Practice brings about change and transformation much more effectively than just thinking about doing something.

Below, slow sex is defined as an actual practice. I have synthesized information from the previous chapters (and cross-referenced it) to explain how to get started in your own personal practice. You can change the guidelines at any time. Feel free to trust your intuition and improvise!

The vital thing is to take it slow, without having great expectations or waiting for a grand display of inner fireworks. Expectations stand in our way of perceiving what actually is; they make us consider what is *not* happening, rather than what *is* happening. Changes are likely to be subtle and gradual, but not necessarily. Great changes can also accompany one single vital insight gained while practicing slow sex. In general, it is a bit like going back to the beginning, being prepared to be an infant again, feeling wobbly and finding a way to walk on two legs, not knowing what's coming next.

The Benefits of a Slow Sex Practice

There are many positive outcomes to the practice of slow sex.

- First and foremost, you become more loving as a human being. Within you lies a deep sense of contentment, of having arrived home, and of self-love. Through the inner connection to yourself the intimacy with the other is deepened.
- There is more harmony and understanding within the relationship, less fighting and controversy between egos, and therefore, fewer emotional ups and downs that disturb love.
- Life seems lighter and much brighter. The sense of well-being deepens. Joy and enjoyment accompany each day.
- Embracing sex in a conscious, slow way is truly transforming and gives rise to deep insights, inspiration, and creativity. When sexual (life) energy is in nature's flow, living gets easier, the outlook is optimistic and positive.
- Reducing the pressure and tension in sex (especially the habit of forcing the body to a climax) boosts the immune system and enhances general health, an effect that becomes more apparent over time.
- The love and awareness generated between two people overflows onto their children and their life as a family unit. The rapport improves and children become more easygoing and self-contained. This relaxation happens because they can sense immediately (and they definitely can, from their earliest moments on Earth) the reassuring fragrance of love in the air.
- Essentially, when a couple decides to be more conscious and

slow in sex they are doing peace work at home, and what they create radiates outward into the world, not only to the immediate family, but also to all those with whom they associate. A couple has the innate power to become tremendous generators of spiritual and positive loving energy in their community.

WHAT KIND OF PRACTICE IS SLOW SEX?

Slow sex can best be described and approached as a loving spiritual practice in which awareness rests in the body and the genitals. We gradually discover how to be present in sex, rather than actively doing sex.

When we have sex with sensitivity and slowness, sex transforms itself into a spiritual practice that creates love and deepens the experience of the present moment.

Any spiritual practice needs to be given time and space in order to feel the benefits. At the same time, even after the first few times you try a more conscious sexual approach, you are quite likely to feel some fulfilling "results," and often in unexpected ways. You may suddenly notice you feel more connected to your partner, more in love (with your partner and yourself), or you feel uplifted and joyful, open, relaxed, and more alive to your senses.

In slow sex practice the attention is rooted in the body generally, and especially in the genital connection—the penis and vagina. Slow sex makes it possible for them to develop their very own language, to exchange energy according to their intrinsic dynamic and receptive qualities. It's a practice that takes time to get the hang of and master, as with any other spiritual practice, or most practices in general. Just as when mastering a musical instrument or a sport, practice and repetition in slow sex lay the foundation for more sustaining and fulfilling experiences.

In certain practices there may be ideals or goals of perfection to be reached, but in slow sex, there are no goals. We immerse ourselves in our bodies and become involved with the unfolding present moment. We see what our bodies want to do, and we watch how they respond intuitively with their own sensual language. We do not interfere and come between the bodies with our minds and preconceived ideas.

At the end of the day, it is ultimately the capacity to turn *inward* that plants in us the roots of our blissful experiences. Bliss and ecstasy do not arrive on demand, but will arise when we give up all mental goals or expectations and relax into a profound acceptance of the body and its inner polarity design. Using the body as a stepping-stone, we can experience the timelessness of the present moment, in which all boundaries evaporate and everything rests in pure peace and harmony.

A Shift in Consciousness, Not a Special Technique

Slow sex is definitely not some kind of special technique, as in a-b-c leads to x-y-z. It is not something that you *do,* but rather something that you become. You enter yourself so as to meet your own body from the inside. Slowing down in sex is based on a shift in consciousness, where the emphasis is on *how* you do something, not *what* you do.

To become slow in sex requires a mental reorientation, a new way of looking at it.

You'll first want to understand the why and the value of trying something new in order to drop or transform the ideas and expectations commonly associated with sex.

Even with good intentions and a fresh orientation, the very first few times you meet you may feel at a bit of a loss as to how to begin. Perhaps you'll even feel a bit confused. This is what happened to me at the outset. I also realized how strange it was that I felt very comfortable with sex when I had a specific and known routine, but as soon as any unknown element entered the picture, I got shaky and unsure of myself. I didn't know who I was, really. When I was relatively unconscious I felt secure, but upon being asked to be a bit more conscious, I felt insecure and thrown into doubt. In reality, feeling confused or insecure is a very natural human response to many situations, so there is absolutely nothing wrong or unusual with any initial hesitation, shyness, or awkwardness.

As much as we live in a society in which sex is very evident in advertising, media, and the like, when it comes down to the reality of this very moment and divesting ourselves of our protection (clothing, the masks of the personality), there can be challenges. You may also feel shy or exposed. But these are not such big hurdles that you need to hold yourself back or prevent yourself from being interested in exploring your higher potential. Confusion and lack of confidence make one feel more vulnerable, open, and present, so any feelings of awkwardness also have positive value. And when feelings are admitted and communicated to the other person in simple words, such as "I feel lost as though I don't know anything anymore," as if giving an inner weather report, then you will immediately feel more relaxed, at ease, and lighthearted. You are being more honest, more authentic, more human. You begin to trust yourself. You will find some more specific suggestions on how to begin later in this chapter.

Slow Sex Is Most Suitable for Long-term Committed Relationships

Our Creator designed human beings for slow sex, so in this sense slow sex is suitable and appropriate for one and all. Simple evolution is available to anyone willing to explore taking sex to another level through being slow. Any person who takes it slow is likely to feel the heightened love and sensitivity that being conscious brings into the exchange, and usually the partner will have a similar experience.

In general, slow sex is most sustainable for heterosexual couples in long-term committed relationships. They have a stable partner with whom to practice over an extended period of time, which is, of course, a great advantage. An opportunity not to take for granted.

> **Many couples eventually are forced to give up having sex for a number of reasons—the most frequent being women's loss of interest or physical discomfort, or male impotence—so slow sex offers a wonderful opportunity to reawaken their sexual life and begin again within a "polarity" framework, a new understanding of the why and how of sex.**

For those couples who are having sex anyway, being conscious and slowing down in sex usually opens the way to a colorful mosaic of experience and expanded love and well-being. A partner is clearly required for the slow sex practice, and at the same time, much can be done as an individual to increase your own awareness and inner sensitivity. As mentioned earlier, inner sex—in which electromagnetic energy streams between the positive and negative poles within your own body—is the most evolved form of sex. Inner sex is valuable whether you are single or in a relationship. At the end of the day you are still a single, in the sense that you are left with yourself and your body. The more interest you invest in exploring your personal inner world, the easier it will be to tune in to the sensitivity called for in slow sex. Many of the exercises in this book are suitable for the individual and can be used as a foundation to grow in awareness and awaken to the cellular light essence of the body.

If you are single and meet someone with whom you wish to be intimate, be alert in your body and senses right from the very first sitting beside each other, bathing in each other's presence, the initial reaching touch, and any ensuing embrace or kiss. This alertness also applies if you are already in a couple and wish to start anew. Begin with being more conscious of what you are doing and how you are doing it. Incorporate awareness into your approach and physical engagement in general, and on each occasion, not just now and then. Small shifts in behavior, such as attempting to pay attention to your own body (and inner body) rather than focusing on your partner's outer body, will usually have a profound impact on the situation. A quality of silence and stillness enters the atmosphere, the senses are alive, and each moment is a jewel to be treasured and valued. Using the awareness in this way (for instance, scanning the body and relaxing tensions, being aware of the breath, relaxing into being rather than doing), you will experience for yourself the positive, transforming, uplifting vibrational influences of the universal metabolic enhancers.

Commitment to the Present Moment

Above all, the personal slow sex journey begins with you and your personal commitment to slow sex. This will be based on your desire, inclination, and willingness to explore new terrain by investigating sexual ways. Transforming or changing old sexual patterns requires a full commitment, not to another person or a relationship, but to oneself. It's not a heavy, burdensome yoke to bear; it's simply the commitment to make a shift, to become aware of what you do and how you do it.

There is an understandable tendency to postpone the sexual investigation for *next* time because you will find (as you have probably already noticed) that as excitement begins to mount, so does the desire for orgasm. That desire and urgency can easily obliterate all alternative intentions, so to make any inroad into the situation you have to take advantage of each and every opportunity presented to you, and not postpone until next time. Deferments will tend to continue, as tomorrow gradually turns into years.

So when can you really start anything at all? Only *now*, and *this* is the moment to begin.

Just a little turn is needed and right around the corner lies the Divine, offering us a new track or direction based on awareness and relaxation andf listening to the intelligence of the body.

Awareness and Vitality
Replace Excitement and Arousal

The great thing about slow sex is that it does not take much energy and you can enter into it even when you are not feeling fresh. It is more a question of whether or not you are able to hold an awareness of the present. Sex can take energy and be arousing at times but does not depend on high energy or getting excited at the outset. It's an engagement with awareness, as has been described in a variety of ways in the previous chapters. Naturally, there will be moments where things will get a bit hotter, but the basic level of arousal (eros) is monitored and intentionally kept cool. At other times, of course, it may be that we get caught up in the excitement and take ourselves to a climax, but with awareness so that these events form part of the experimentation.

The significant thing is to do whatever you do with awareness. Nothing is implicitly wrong in orgasm; it's just the habit of running toward it and the tension that is built up to achieve it that is being questioned.

You attempt to relax into the orgasm. Avoid becoming too tense and focused on the destination, but instead find a way to arrive there at a more leisurely pace. Using the universal metabolic enhancers in this way will transform the situation into something fresh and innocent.

GETTING STARTED AT YOUR SLOW SEX PRACTICE

Here I offer some specific pointers that may be useful as you begin to transform your sexual practice into a spiritually uplifting exchange. Pointers include information on preparation and foreplay, how to make and keep a sustained connection, physical penetration with or without erection, and how to conclude a slow sex encounter and resume other activities.

Make a Date to Make Love

We make dates and appointments for countless things, why not for sex? Human beings don't have enough sustainable and fulfilling sex, so setting a fixed time makes absolute sense. In fact, the best way to establish slow sex as a sustainable practice is to set aside times specifically for that purpose. It's of great value to establish a regular place and time for slow sex. Plan it and incorporate it into your life just as you would a yoga practice or any exercise regimen. Choose a date, choose a time, choose a venue. Sit down together and decide, and then write SS down on your weekly calendar. And from then onward, on a week-by-week basis, intentionally create space and make dates for sex. Just as we prioritize certain other activities, we can bring slow sex into the foreground and give human union a higher value.

Dedicating time to sex usually means that you will have to make fewer appointments with friends and family. You will also need to make appropriate arrangements if you have children at home, so that they will be looked after or kept otherwise engaged. Remember that love made between a couple radiates outward onto the children, so children should never be used as an excuse not to make time for slow sex. Be certain to switch off all phones and cellular devices so you can enjoy tranquility and peace without any interruptions or disturbances.

Creating a protected or sacred space leads to a deeper level of relaxation, awareness, and sensitivity. By making a date for sex you make yourselves available to each other; sex is not happening by accident, habit, or routine, or not at all! Instead the meeting and joining is a conscious choice by two consenting and willing people wishing to commune sexually with each other on a spiritual level. The intention behind the sexual meeting will automatically elevate the ensuing experience. You know what you are doing and why you are doing it.

Starting out with a fixed appointment might initially feel a bit unromantic or clinical, but once you get accustomed to it, these conscious meetings feel ordinary and completely natural.

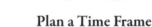

Plan a Time Frame
That Is Realistic and Sustainable

There are no rules about how much time to devote to sex. What you can manage is what you can manage, and at the same time a certain level of commitment is required. Anywhere upward of forty-five minutes is advisable. When at all possible, try to give yourselves a basic minimum of three hours, because it does require time to warm up and enter fully into the situation. This is not necessarily true for men, but is certainly true for women, because female sexual energy takes longer to awaken. This difference in sexual temperatures and readiness is the vital difference between men and women, as explained in detail in chapter 5. When the underlying polarity difference is acknowledged and embraced, sexual communion is easily elevated; there is a shift that leads to a finer tuning. And when man understands that the more open woman is, the higher he himself will be able to fly, he is more than willing to grant woman what she needs.

At the start of our retreats we tell couples that they will be given a three-hour window for slow sex each and every day. Most of them look quite aghast and shy; disbelieving laughter usually ripples around the room. Within a handful of days, however, many are happily and confidently announcing that three hours are simply not enough. These don't have to be three hours of solid lovemaking, although this may certainly happen on occasion. At any time during slow sex you can simply stop (by mutual decision, or sharing your needs) to drink a cup of tea, take a shower, go to the toilet, change the music, adjust your positions, or whatever. And then afterward, you return to bed and begin again.

Each time will have its own flavor and fragrance. That's the beauty of slow sex—you never know how it's going to be. There's no set routine; it's always an unfolding according to the constellation of the moment and the presence and awareness of the parties involved.

Two hours, one hour, or half an hour will be fine if that is all you can accommodate. Periodically it is really worthwhile to give yourselves a whole day in bed, eating and showering and refreshing yourselves as needed, but continually going back to bed, lying around, cuddling and snuggling. The more you make yourselves available for experience, the more surprising, spontaneous, graceful, and flowing the bodies become— joining in relaxation and ease.

The slow sex approach includes a version of the famous conventional sexual quickie, too. Does this surprise you? Remember that slow sex is all about *how* you do something more than *what* you do. So the slow sex quickie is a conscious, harmonizing get-together or gentle congress for some minutes, anywhere from ten or fifteen to forty-five, depending on your time frame. The quickie is a gentle fusion of the genitals as described in chapter 4, in the section on soft entry without the need for erection and excitement. If there is arousal and erection, you penetrate extremely slowly, then just flow with or be with what is present.

A quickie suits occasions when there is not as much time as you'd like, but ten or fifteen minutes is feasible. Quickies can be enjoyed any time of the day—morning, afternoon, evening, or all of the above. Mornings are a perfect time to come home to yourself and anchor yourself in your inner reality before you engage with the outer world; this simple type of energy exchange has a subtle yet profound impact on the quality of your day. You will feel more positive, more alert, more alive, more happy. Quickies are also perfect for afternoon siesta hours, and a quickie at night can help send you off to a more peaceful sleep.

Frequency of Slow Sex Appointments

Slow sex needs to take place on a relatively regular basis if there is a wish to develop more sensitivity and experience its beneficial rewards. Two or three or four times a week is good, and every day is, of course, the optimum.

> **The more loving sex we have, the more we wish for it. The more we practice, the more insights we receive, the more we learn and understand.**

If we don't make love often enough it is easy for complacency and laziness to overshadow our good intentions, as we forget the positive effects of slow sex and how inwardly uplifted, more connected to our partner, and appreciative of life it makes us feel.

As far as regularity goes, maintaining the same time of day every day (or on designated days) will make it easier to sustain a slow sex practice. And any time of the day or night is suitable—dawn, morning, afternoon, sunset, and moonlit midnight are all perfect times. Each part of the day brings its own quality, and experimenting with time of the day or night will introduce more variety and spontaneity into the exchange. It may be easier to be fully present at certain times of the day or night, so decide on a time that works well for both of you. Personally, I have always favored mornings and fortunately my flexible schedule allows for this. It's a juicy and inspiring way to start the day! I find my mind more empty (less cluttered by daily thoughts), my body more fresh and open, and it's easier to fall into the innocence of being. Some men may prefer mornings as well, because at that time of day testosterone levels are said to be higher, which is something to consider if there is difficulty getting an erection. However, the option of entry without erection makes union possible at any time.

Impotence Poses No Barrier to Slow Sex

Many aspects of impotence have their basis in man's mind. Often man equates or identifies his ability to achieve an erection with basic manhood, so when erection is lost he feels so insecure and unworthy that his whole identity can crumble. Without a hard penis, who am I?

When the causes of impotence are understood (as an excess of stimulation leading to loss of sensitivity and numbing of tissues and nerve responses), then a doorway is opened for great healing, penis rebalancing, and a slow style of sexual interchange that is based on sensitivity and not sensation. Impotence is not a dead-end road, as most people imagine or experience. I heard on television the other day that an estimated twenty million men today are regularly taking Viagra! This is a sad situation. It's sad that so many men have erection disturbances (and certainly there are more who are not taking Viagra), but also, Viagra serves only to satisfy man's mind (not the body, the body is simply used). Viagra fulfills the man's psychological need to experience himself as virile and hard, even if it's chemically orchestrated. The body is simply used as a vehicle to satisfy one of the deepest insecurities in a man—the fear of losing erection and not feeling like a real man.

From the slow sex perspective, true male authority arises through man's capacity to be present to himself and his penis, and present to woman when he is inside her, and has nothing to do with erection per se.

In these circumstances erection or half erection may spontaneously arise (even when man is reportedly impotent) because the interplay of dynamic and receptive forces creates the erection. Not stimulation. A magnetism arises within and between the bodies. Certainly men who have shared about their Viagra experiences with me are aware that its main value is psychological—they say having a hard-on gives self-confidence, a sense of self. At the same time, I have also been told that when using Viagra the sensitivity of the penis is not particularly enhanced, that there is not that much genuine feeling. I also understand that sometimes the erection continues after sex is over—it just won't go down and can sometimes become painful or disturbing for the man.

Preparing the Sacred Space

As a venue for slow sex your own bedroom is perfect. If you have an extra room in your house, you may want to turn it into a love temple—specifically reserved.

- You'll need a big comfortable bed and privacy. Sometimes couples will move their bedroom furniture around and clear away clutter so as to create more space and a fresh awareness of their surroundings.
- Many couples buy a new mattress. The comfort of the bed is vital if you are to spend many hours in it beyond your usual sleeping hours. A large bed with a relatively firm and supportive mattress is best. Mattresses that are too soft cause the bodies to roll toward the middle (which means the mattress gives no support), and the changing of positions and so on becomes more awkward and cumbersome.
- Do not restrict yourselves to beds, either. Sofas, tables, and the floor also offer suitable places for bodies in semi- and fully horizontal positions.
- Make your room beautiful by adding flowers, lighting candles, and spraying fragrance.
- Lighting can play a significant part in creating atmosphere. Use well-placed lamps in corners of the room, for example. Some level of lighting is necessary in the sense that you want to be able to see your partner's eyes and face. Sex in the dark can also be magical sometimes, but you'll mostly want to maintain contact with your partner's eyes. Soft, receptive eyes are also a significant tool for remaining in the present.
- Music is enjoyed and valued by lovers because of its powerfully enveloping qualities that help us to relax into our bodies, enter the present, and go with the flow. At the same time, and depending on the piece of music selected, it is pos-

sible for a person to get carried away with the intensity of the music, slip out of awareness, and get caught up in making something happen. As the music gets more dramatic you may also get more dramatic. Experiment with music and no music, and observe its impact on you. Choose music that does not carry you away, but helps you to be present. Don't use music as a habit or crutch; from time to time allow yourselves to be surrounded by sounds of silence or nature, or whatever other sounds are present in the environment.

Preparation and Foreplay

When you look at your calendar on the agreed-upon day and see the 8 p.m. to 11 p.m. date scheduled, you are likely to inwardly notice a smile and feel the thrill of joy and anticipation. The "knowing" can act as a kind of a subtle foreplay that inwardly prepares you for the meeting. Throughout the day you can begin to tune in to your body, especially for man in the perineum, and for woman in the breasts and nipples. These are the poles that raise male and female sexual energy, so it builds energy and vitality if you maintain an awareness in these places. Again and again, go to these places and infuse them with your breath and your awareness, as if touching and massaging yourself on the inside.

Connecting to your body and feeling alive and well in your own physical being will enhance the experience.

Sex takes place between two bodies, so begin by entering your own body with awareness and connecting with your inner aliveness.

Your increased inner vitality will have a big impact on your sensitivity and capacity to be present. You may want to take a luxurious warm bath followed by a cold shower, do some kind of exercise that you enjoy, dance a wild dance, massage yourself or exchange massage, sing a few songs, shake for fifteen minutes, maintain conscious breathing, or lie down and tune in to yourself. Anything will do, really. The idea is to channel your awareness into your body and there are a variety of ways to do so. Ritual and prayer can also be used as powerful forms of preparation to harmonize the energy and enter the present. It is not absolutely essential to prepare every time, but good to realize that preparation makes it much easier to tune in and come alive to the vibrant inner realms of the body.

Tools, Not Rules

There are definitely no rules about how to practice; just follow your feelings or intuition in each situation. Be guided by your body and listen to its gentle whispers. If you feel a spontaneous urge or pull arising from your body, follow it, flow with it. Don't hold yourself back with the thought that this is not how it is meant to be. If you hold back for even a couple of seconds the moment will be lost, the wave you might have ridden has passed through you and is now beyond reach. Any time I ever repressed myself in that way I was always the loser. Learn to trust the body and surrender to its language and undulating expression.

All the suggestions throughout this book are designed to help you keep your attention anchored in the present, to stay aware of what is taking place in each and every moment. The most significant aspect is that whatever you choose to do, you do with awareness; that is all. The guidelines offered are merely tools that can help you root yourself in your body, which is a prerequisite for experiencing slowness in sex.

HOW TO PROCEED—GETTING YOUR FIRST SLOW SEX DATE OFF THE GROUND

Here you are on your very first slow sex date and it is finally time to put theory into practice. For some of you, slow sex comes easily, almost as if it's your second nature. It is! You find it simple to enter into a shared awareness and fall into a sensuous, non-goal-oriented exploration in which you relate to each other's bodies in a relaxed, easy way. If this is the case for you and your partner, just keep trusting your bodies doing whatever they're doing, always being mindful to keep a clear, cool, and conscious connection alive between you.

For others, and perhaps for most, the first slow sex encounter is going to be a bit awkward. You may even feel embarrassed or shy, at a loss for what's supposed to happen next. This is to be expected. How can one know a language fluently without going through a period of practice, which includes much trial and error? It's important to give yourselves a big time frame, not to try slowness just once or twice. If it's difficult for any reason, people will tend to revert to their more familiar, tried-and-true sexual behaviors. The known becomes very attractive because it's a sexual "comfort zone" and it's not so comfortable to feel uncomfortable—at any time really, but particularly in sex where the ego is very identified with a certain sexual style.

At the end of some preceding chapters there are specific exercises designed to support you, as individuals and as a couple. Some are exercises to practice alone (although you can do them in the company of your partner, both perhaps doing the same thing simultaneously), while other exercises are shared experiences. Practicing any of these will direct you to the delights of your inner world and help you be more present in your body and present in the situation. That basic shift back to yourself is all you need to begin your slow sex practice. For convenience, the exercises are also described below (in somewhat less detail), which means that some repetition of suggestions is unavoidable.

Making the Inner Connection

The very first step is to make contact with yourself, within your own body. Sex happens between two bodies, so this initial step is more significant than having immediate contact with your partner. To get closer to another person you must first get closer to yourself—and literally closer to your very own body. Enter into the world of your inner body where the source of cellular sensitivity and aliveness lies. The awareness rises in your body before you begin thinking about, or turning toward, your partner. What follows with your partner flows and evolves from your initial inner connection. In fact, your inner rootedness makes it very simple to establish contact with the other person. You feel more confident and you trust yourself. The essential inner connection can be made by practicing the following exercise.

☽ Exercise: Finding Home in Your Body

You can either practice this exercise alone before you meet with your partner or you and your partner can do the exercise together as a way to begin your slow sex date.

1. If you and your partner are doing the exercise together, sit, stand, or lie opposite each other and a little apart, without physical contact.
2. Close your eyes gently and take two or three easy, full breaths through the diaphragm and into your belly. Scan your body and relax any part that's holding tension.
3. Then each of you should take your attention inward and downward into your own body and look for a place that feels like a "home" in the body. It might be the heart, solar plexus, low back, belly, feet, genitals, or wherever—anywhere below the head—that will internally connect you to the realms of your flesh, blood, and bones.

An inner home acts as a resting place, a connection point, working like an anchor that holds your attention within the body. When you have made this inner connection you'll be more ready to open your eyes and meet the eyes of your partner.

Making Eye Contact with Your Partner

In slow sex, learning to keep soft, receptive eye contact with your partner becomes an important tool for deepening your connection to each other, while at the same time staying centered in your own body. The following exercise will give you some pointers on how to develop this skill.

☺ Exercise: Practicing Soft Vision with Your Partner

1. When you feel rooted within your body, you can begin to open your eyes fraction by fraction (without losing contact with your inner body—if you do lose this connection, please close your eyes again until you inwardly reconnect).

2. When your eyes are fully open, gently meet your partner's eyes. Allow your partner into you through the eyes. Let your eyes be gentle, soft, receptive, and inviting. It will be easier to gaze receptively at just one of your partner's eyes at a time.

3. Take a deep breath into your belly and let your eyes receive what is there in front of them, rather than looking outward in an objective or judgmental fashion.

4. Continue to breathe deeply, relaxing the belly, and softening the muscles surrounding the genitals. Be present in your body, simple and innocent.

5. Remain in receptive eye sharing mode for as long as it feels comfortable, and close the eyes whenever it feels necessary, either to reconnect inwardly or to sense yourself even more deeply on the inside. Keep coming back to open eyes and being available to yourself on the inside as you receive your partner's soft gaze into you. Avoid keeping the eyes closed for extended periods.

This special soft and receptive way of using the eyes has the advantage of enabling you to connect with your partner and, at the same time, keep your attention on the inside of yourself. Your attention within your own body can be seen as your priority. You embrace, kiss, and make love with the body, so there has to be some sort of process to enter into it. If and when the inner connection is lost (which can easily happen at first), simply close your eyes again and relax back into your body, retreating into the suggested "home." Open your eyes again when you feel more rooted in yourself.

The First Physical Contact with Your Partner

When you get the feeling of being able to stay with yourself on the inside, and at the same time be open to your partner on the outside (and this may require practice), then you can move consciously across the space separating you and generously extend your arms or your hand or your lips, moving into whatever contact feels right in the moment—an embrace, touching and caressing with sensitive hands, or a kiss that is sustained by keeping the lips soft, relaxed, and sealed together.

Avoid choosing a position that is your habitual cuddle position, because it's already so familiar to you both that it won't be easy for you to feel any difference or make any difference. For instance, a woman should keep her head straight when embracing a man, instead of turning it to the side and resting it cosily on his shoulder or chest. When the head, neck, and spine are in one line, it's easier to turn the awareness inward. Physically you are further away from your partner, but you will feel yourself more present and more connected energetically. Likewise, a man should not collapse forward over his woman during an embrace, but keep an alignment through head, neck, and spine. If a man is much taller than his woman, he can stand with his legs wide astride so as to lower his height, rather than bend forward over the woman. Or the woman can stand on a stable cushion, or on a step to increase her height. Standing on tiptoes can work, but it is not easy to sustain for longer periods.

Another Way to Begin:
Establish Polarity within Yourself

All human beings have an internal magnet within, with a positive pole at one end and a negative pole at the other. Woman's positive pole is her breasts. Man's positive pole is his penis. When each partner brings their own positive pole to life before the individual bodies move together, the meeting will be filled with a special circular energy.

☺ Exercise: Establishing Personal Polarity before First Contact

1. Stand or lie down without physical contact, three or four feet apart.

2. Close your eyes and take up an inner connection with yourself. Take the time to drop within and establish yourself in your inner body.

3. Then, after some minutes, man places his attention on the perineum (the area at the root of the penis in front of the anus) and woman places her attention on her nipples. The idea is not to concentrate or focus on these parts, but to melt into them and bring them to life. Visualize the tissues filling with love, light, and vitality.

4. Take some time, and when you have the feeling of being connected with yourself, alive to yourself, turn gradually toward each other and, inch by conscious inch, close the space separating you, bringing the bodies into their first contact.

5. Don't push your bodies into each other in a hard physical way; let there be some inches of space between you so that contact is porous and fluffy and ensures that the energy bodies remain vibrant and expanded.

6. In your own time move ever so slowly into an embrace or kiss (or whatever) with eyes closed or open, whatever feels right.

Some Alternative Approaches

Another approach is to lie (or stand) with your bodies several feet apart, and before you physically connect, allow your eyes to meet for several minutes in a receptive vision connection, as described earlier. Or man can gently lay his hands on woman's breasts while she gently lays her cupped hand over his pubic mound and penis. Or the testicles can be gently lifted from beneath and held warmly and lovingly in the hand.

The orientation is toward aliveness and awareness rather than stimulation and excitement. You are looking for what helps to open and expand your partner's energy field, rather than what turns them (or you) on and causes the energy field to contract.

This is a basic guideline for any type of foreplay, that it should lead toward sensitivity and *expansion* of energy rather than excitement and *contraction* of energy, which can easily give rise to restlessness and the desire to go after orgasm.

THE FIRST SLOW SEX PENETRATION

It is possible that your very first date or dates will not progress as far as actual sex, so it is important to keep pace with what unfolds and feels comfortable for you both, rather than feel compelled to get somewhere specific. A childlike, innocent approach is a great support. If and when you feel ready to get your bodies together, then you can do so in ways described below, or follow your intuition.

There are two basic scenarios that you are likely to be presented with: when man has an erection and when he does not. So man should not be overly concerned about his erection. If it's there, you enter woman in one way; if it's not there, you enter in another way.

At this stage or at any earlier point, you can both oil or lubricate your own genitals, or each other's, bearing in mind the touch must not be a very stimulating one. Lubrication is covered in more detail in chapter 4; it is really helpful if you use lubrication every time you make love.

With Erection:
Make the Initial Penetration Exceptionally Slow

The value of an exceptionally slow entry into woman's body is described earlier in chapter 4, and is particularly significant for women if they are virgins, and also later in menopausal years. When man enters woman slowly (and with lubrication), she usually will not feel pain because man is being conscious and honoring her receptive feminine environment. The missionary position is perhaps the most suitable for slow penetration, but it can also be done in the side-scissors position and a number of other positions. In missionary position, woman can place a thick flat pillow under her buttocks to raise her pelvis and bring the vagina closer to the penis (see fig. 10.1).

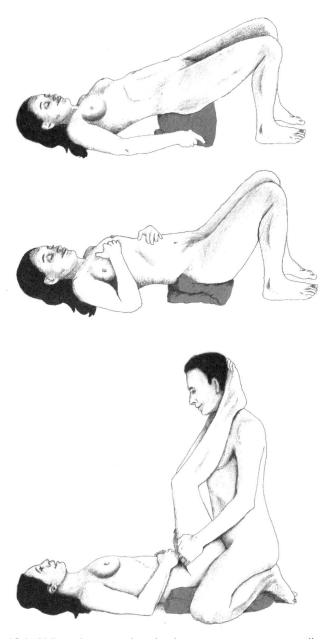

Fig. 10.1. When lying on her back, woman can use a pillow support under the buttocks to raise the level of her pelvis. In the first image woman uses her legs to raise her pelvis and place the pillow in position. Its final position is shown in the second image. The third image shows a nice variation of the missionary position with woman's feet resting on man's shoulders.

◎ Slow Penetration Step by Step

Step one: Woman must spread her lips and can keep her hands there for some time while holding the lips apart. This clearing of the pathway allows for unimpeded penetration, graceful and highly pleasurable, especially when lubrication is used. Opening the lips will bring crystal clarity into the contact and heighten the correspondence between the dynamic pole (penis) and the receptive pole (vagina). At a certain point woman may have to move her hands away because they no longer fit between the pelvises, however I strongly recommend that woman repeat this spreading action of the lips frequently during the union, and not be shy about doing so. Man will need to pull back a few inches to allow space for woman's hands, but the slight interruption has great rewards in terms of thrilling magnetic contact.

Step two: The next step is for man to place the head of the penis at the entrance of the vagina and wait for a few moments. Then you can make eye contact in a gentle way and, should you wish to, you can maintain eye contact for the duration.

Step three: And then man can, literally millimeter by millimeter, begin to glide in with utter consciousness, the focus of his awareness in the perineum as well as the head of the penis. Be aware that if woman feels the penis is entering her too fast or without a loving awareness, she will unconsciously (or consciously) tighten the vagina to prohibit deeper entry.

Stop along the way and feel the moment, as if you are pausing on a riverside walk and appreciating the waterfalls, the damp air, the silver bubbles, the silently streaming undercurrent. Slow sex enjoys and values the immediate present, what is happening for real, and not what the mind thinks should happen. The journey has a variety of moments along the way, and there is no real final destination in mind. The first (or any) penetration can last several minutes (or hours), and the penis can remain in the glory of the depths of the vagina (provided this is comfortable for woman; if not, please see chapter 8 on pain and the healing or purification of the genitals). There is no need to regularly move in and out of the vagina. When the moment feels right, all moves within the vagina should be done with consciousness and slowness. In general, rapid, friction-oriented movements are avoided, as these cause woman to shrink on a subtle level, lose her receptivity, and lead in exciting directions instead.

Through using the awareness the immediate instant is highlighted and you will find yourselves slipping into another realm, one in which you are invisibly yet powerfully connected to some higher force. You become totally engaged in, and utterly enthralled by, each and every moment. Seconds effortlessly roll into hours of flowing beauty and grace.

There should be no attempt to keep the erection going; if it fades away, then relax down into the side-scissors position (see fig. 10.2) and remain in genital union.

Without Erection: Connect Using Soft Entry

Soft penetration is suitable if there is no erection, and has been described in detail in chapter 4. Soft penetration is a perfectly valid way to begin. In fact, for many couples starting out soft becomes their standard way. From there many things can happen, including erection, but erection per se loses its significance. In fact, my lover and I had the curious experience over many years that he would usually go in soft to start and come out hard when we had finished. Everything turns on its head when the approach to sex is simplified. Obsessions and insecurities about the need for erection gradually fade, for both man and woman, and are replaced by the simplicity and innate sensitivity of the genital connection.

☉ Soft Penetration Step by Step

Woman can help a man to enter her, and some positions are particularly suited for soft penetration, such as the so-called side-scissors position, shown on page 124. This is a position in which both partners can be physically comfortable for an extended period and it lends itself to relaxed nondoing because neither partner is on top.

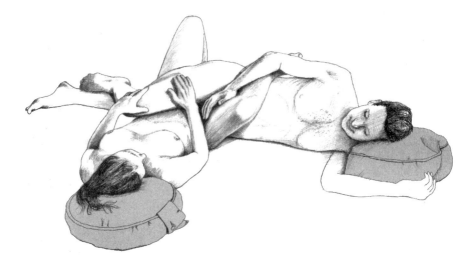

Fig. 10.2. In side-scissors position woman lies on her back
and man lies on his side, their legs intertwined in a
scissors-like fashion. Head support for both partners,
as shown here, is helpful for sustained relaxation.

Step one: When you are both in position the very first thing a woman should do is open the vaginal lips by moving them aside to expose the vaginal entrance.

Step two: Then woman can reach behind the head of the penis, taking it between the index and third finger with a gentle yet firm squeeze.

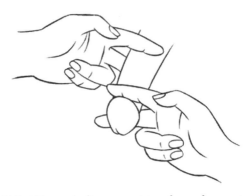

Fig. 10.3. Woman's finger position for soft penetration

Step three: Then she lies down on her back (to keep belly relaxed and vagina open) and guides the head toward the vaginal entrance pushing the first inch or so into the vagina; even just the head is enough to start. With a little dexterity, practice, and moving the fingers back a few centimeters, step-by-step the rest of the penis can be fed into the vagina.

Step four: Then relax back into yourselves, keeping awareness on the genital connection, breathing slowly and deeply and maintaining eye contact—not as a rule, but as a tool. You may want to close them now and then, perhaps to sink more fully into yourself.

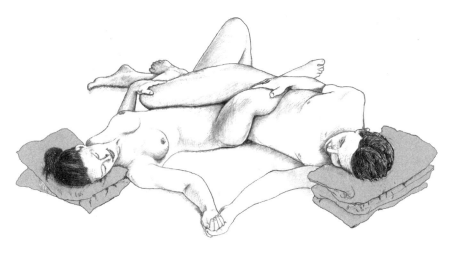

Fig. 10.4. In a nice variation on side-scissors position man and woman can hold hands and gaze softly into each other's eyes.

The side-scissors position is just a start and has value because both partners can relax simultaneously. However, you can alter your position at any time, according to what is needed. For example, if erection arises spontaneously, you may wish to adjust position to be more present and involved. Or you may feel movement will disturb what is taking place.

FINISH SLOW SEX
BY RETURNING TO YOURSELF

Couples often tell us that once they get the knack of slow sex they sometimes find it surprisingly difficult to stop. And they ask us, "How do you, in fact, stop?" Indeed, in the beginning it can feel a bit strange to complete sex without having a climax to mark the end. An orgasm functions like a full stop at the end of a flowing sentence. However, once you become more accustomed to it, not "finishing" feels normal and not unusual in any way at all. We usually reply to such questions by explaining that you have to be practical. If you need to go somewhere or do something, then you must; just be sure to separate as you have been together—with awareness. So you simply disconnect the genitals and bodies gently and gracefully, bowing to each other, or find a way that completes the union for you.

Then take a few minutes to lie on your back and dive into your own body again, bringing all the wonder back home to yourself as an individual. I was interested to hear from a participant recently about the magnetic fields that surround a person because he had the capacity to measure such energies using a pendulum. He measured his own and his girlfriend's individual magnetic radiance prior to making love. And then he measured them while joined in sex and established that the magnetic field was greatly increased—and much larger than the sum total of their two individual fields. Then afterward, when they were physically separated, he discovered that each individual had retained the larger magnetic field. In union they become one large field, and in separation two identical twin energy fields remained. Fascinating!

I have always found it very important to finish a slow sex encounter by coming back to myself before leaping out of bed and getting involved in the next steps required of me. If I leave the sacred space of awareness too quickly, later I find I sometimes feel a bit wobbly, fragile, or oversensitive (slightly emotional—see later in the section on issues that may arise). If there is no real or urgent need to stop having sex, then don't! Why on Earth stop having sex? The bodies will naturally come to an easy completion in due course. When the bodies become fully engaged and get on a roll of their own, spectacular moments unfold between you, and before you know it you have been plugged in for hours on end.

How you finish is as important as how you start. Separate consciously, disconnect slowly, and come back to yourself and into your own space for several minutes.

Usually it is quite nice to have a period without physical contact so that you can reconnect with yourself as an individual. Lie down or sit and be with yourself, attention in the body and being present to the delicate sensations now streaming within you. Take fifteen or twenty minutes. If you disconnect too quickly and run off to do some urgent task, then you may later start to swing the other way. After an experience of expansion in consciousness it is good and appropriate to ground the experience in your own body, so that the opposite swing is not encouraged. When you take time for yourself and remain present in the awareness, there is a natural balancing force to any swings, and you are less likely to feel disoriented or vulnerable.

SUSTAINING YOUR SLOW SEX PRACTICE

Like any practice, slow sex needs to be sustained for a good period of time in order to reap its benefits and transformative powers. This means that to keep your slow sex commitment alive, you'll want to make dates to meet as often as possible. Below are some guidelines to keep you on track, comfortable, and curious in your exploration. Sometimes people say that the journey looks long and arduous, and wonder how long it will take to get there. The truth is that you never get anywhere! You only get more and more here. And this cannot be a goal because your body is *already* here. It's more a matter of appreciating your here-ness, getting your mind to pay attention to your body in the present moment, feeling rather than thinking, and generally shifting your perception from the outer to the inner.

For me personally, there has never been any resistance, conflict, or difficulty, and perhaps that is so because I have had absolutely no goal or objective all along. I have not tried to get anywhere or achieve anything. My intention at the outset and in my early thirties was to change the way I made love. As simple as that. No big theories. And not because I was dissatisfied or bored, not in the slightest. Just inquisitive. Actually at that time, in the situation in which I was living, there was an abundance of possible sex partners and many flavors to enjoy. I began out of sheer curiosity to know more about my body. I connected with one man in particular and we started from zero, from where we were, and that is pretty much the same place for each one of us—conditioned to have fast sex with orgasm as a focus.

My exploration brought me many understandings and insights. It's not that I knew all I know and understand today at the outset. Not at all. I was totally innocent in that sense. Clarity arises, insights descend, sensitivity increases, heart expands, body balances—all as by-products of practice, not as prerequisites to it. That is why I insist that slow sex is not a technique, it is not something you do and follow like a recipe, instead it evolves steadily.

Slow sex is something you enter and become, an ambience that you create through your bodily relaxation, awareness, and presence, and you change as a result. Profound personal transformation is possible simply by changing the way you have sex, shifting from being unconscious to conscious.

Sex lies at the foundation of our system, the lowest major energy center. Any shifts and changes in the base will definitely ripple throughout and have an impact on the higher energy centers that lie above.

To encourage couples I sometimes tell them the truth about myself, that I am basically a very lazy person. And the only, and I mean only, reason that I am in a position to sit in front of them and share my experience with them is because everything happened lying down. I was comfortably horizontal in bed, so for me it was pure heaven. If it had been necessary to do the whole exploration in a standing posture, then I can say with certainty that I would not be in a position to say anything about sex today.

Remaining Present in the Sexual Encounter

To be in the present means to include any aspect of the metabolic enhancers as outlined in the previous chapters, such as awareness, rhythm, and relaxation—there are many subtle ways for you to remain present. For example, using awareness you can travel internally to different parts of the body—man might want to travel to his positive pole in the perineum, woman to her nipples. You can also experiment with relaxing other parts of the body—man, the anus and buttocks; woman, the vagina, and anywhere else too. Stay here and now with the unfolding moment, alert in your senses, aware in your body, playful and curious.

- Relax your body consciously again and again, scanning from head to toe, looking for tense places, relaxing and letting go. Release the unconscious holding in the shoulders, the jaw, the solar plexus, the belly, and the muscles around the genitals. Each time you intentionally relax your body you may notice that a spontaneous deep breath follows, along with a wave of subtle sensation moving through your cells.
- Engage each other's eyes as much as possible, with inviting vision, so most of your awareness remains rooted within your own body. Close your eyes when you feel the need to sink deeper into yourself. Speak about your wishes to your partner. This avoids giving them the impression that you are escaping the situation or somehow abandoning them. Sharing helps you to avoid possible misunderstandings.

- Keep your attention on your breathing. Breathe deeply and slowly. Breathe into the diaphragm and belly, imagine your breath touching the genitals. Breathing is a simple bridge that can lead you from thinking to a greater immersion in the body. Breathe in and out together, or one person breathes in as the other breathes out. These breathing patterns will often establish themselves on their own, but it's good to explore the effects of doing them deliberately.
- Kissing, caressing, and touching all keep us present in our bodies and senses. Touch consciously and without any demand, just a loving, generous touch.
- Smile a little, keep your lip corners up, and observe what doing that does to your facial feeling and present moment.

Notice how these small offerings, as acts of awareness, can weave together to become a significant contribution to the intricate tapestry.

Share the Experience of Your Now

The present moment can be greatly magnified by sharing what you are experiencing within yourself, how you feel on a heart level, and any subtle sensations and sensitivities you might be experiencing on a body level. Letting your partner know what you are feeling and where you are feeling it opens a window into your inner realms. Sharing literally brings you into a shared world, which is very helpful at the outset as you establish an unfamiliar style of sex. It's good to know what's going on inside each other. Otherwise you are both left guessing, which may give rise to doubts and tension, and these would not help or support your exploration.

On the other hand, just a few words reporting what you feel can be tremendously relaxing for you and your partner. Share small observations in a few words: "I feel a tingling" (or warmth, light, or whatever it is you happen to feel). Inner sensations are continually changing, shifting, moving, flowing, streaming, so there is usually something small to observe and share. No big discussion and your partner does not need to respond in any way, other than to also say what he or she is feeling at the time.

Extraordinarily, when inner cellular sensations are acknowledged, they amplify. Just by bringing attention to good feelings or good places in the body they will immediately respond by expanding.

When you tell someone about your inner experience, you are simultaneously communicating this to your body, your higher self, and especially to your brain, and this is very powerful. Speaking out reeducates you making you more conscious, more here, and more alert.

⌒

Give Space to Feelings that Arise

There is much pain and sadness associated with sex, either from personal experiences in the past or from collective pain due to the misunderstanding, abuse, and repression that has happened through conventional sex. Every individual has felt the impact of these pressures and tensions to a greater or lesser degree, whether we know it or not. It's in the atmosphere, and from our very earliest months of life we are affected by what we feel, sense, see, hear, touch, and imagine. We are shaped by invisible forces; there is no choice, it's a conditioning that grows in us unconsciously. It's a twist on the sexual picture that causes us to lose touch with our sexual innocence, our conscious nature, our restful beings, our loving hearts. Therefore, when consciousness enters the sexual frame, it is a deeply healing force that will begin to move unhappiness out of the system, so it is quite usual for tears to flow. It's a really positive response and highly beneficial to let tears move through you and out of you. In this sense, be open to yourself and yield to your tears, pain, or whatever comes up for you.

If you feel or sense nothing in particular in your genitals, and this is very common at the outset, say so. And also share how it feels not to feel. Admitting to this is taking a big step toward regaining your lost sensitivity. If suddenly tears begin to flow, let them flow; they will refresh your heart. Afterward, you will most probably observe an increase in sensitivity and an aliveness in your cells, especially in the penis or vagina.

When you observe the sensations of a rising feeling—and are able to catch it in the split second it arises—stay with the sensation and open a passage for it. Surrender to it and give way to the flow. Don't hold back or repress for an instant. When you stay faithful to a rising feeling you will often notice that it lasts only seven seconds or so. It passes through you like a wave, and afterward you feel more alive and open.

When buried things are on the move it's usually impossible to communicate to your partner what is happening without stopping the feelings or distancing you from them. At the same time, sometimes saying a word or two, admitting to yourself and thereby your partner, can initiate a healthy torrent of feelings, and it's cleansing to let whatever comes up emerge. Otherwise these feelings remain in the body and are stored as emotions, which generally numb and desensitize the system and also revisit us in destructive and habitual ways (see later section: "Separating Love from Emotion").

Giving free yet conscious rein to your withheld or repressed feelings is profoundly healing and refreshing, both physically and spiritually.

You may also experience unstoppable laughter from time to time, or uncontrollable shaking and shivering, or sadness and tears may reach deeper into heart-wrenching sobbing and wailing. You do not have to understand why you are weeping and wailing or whatever, just live it. Insights as to why may come, or they may not. But don't waste or miss healing opportunities by trying to analyze and figure out why this is happening to you. It is happening, so welcome it; don't try to control it through analysis.

Anger can also come up during sex, in both men and women.

Anger has certain golden rules attached to it and these rules
must be obeyed at all costs.

Do not project your anger onto your partner. Immediately turn to the side and away from your partner before you let the wave of rage or frustration pass through, perhaps in one grand roar. Or leap out of bed and begin jumping up and down on flat feet, heels hitting the floor first. Keep the arms raised and shout out "Ho!" each time you land on your heels. Do this for several minutes until the wave of anger has passed. The source of all anger lies in accumulated sexual frustration, and most humans are frustrated sexually in the sense that we have not experienced ourselves as a unit of dynamic/receptive forces with an inherent circular movement between man and woman, fulfilling a divine cycle of giving and receiving. So it is very common to feel anger, even rage, arise during sex; take it as an encouraging sign that anger has risen as a way to purify the cells.

Changing and Holding Positions with Awareness

There are no special positions other than the ones that work for you and your partner. It is awareness that makes a position valid and valuable, and not the position per se. It's good to change positions. Once you have achieved genital union you can change position at any time to refresh yourself and become more alert to the situation. Positions and their significance were discussed in chapter 4, where figures 4.5 and 4.6 illustrate the two sequences of rotating positions that allow movement while the penis remains within the vagina (or if not, slip it back in). Or there are some positions that can be held for a longer time without much movement. The side-scissors position is particularly good for sustained penetration with or without erection. (See figs. 10.6 and 10.7 on pages 139 and 140, which illustrate some props that can make the position even more comfortable.)

Yab yum (fig. 10.5 on page 134) is a really wonderful position because

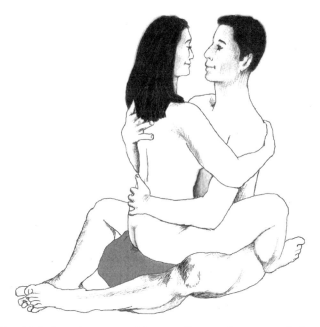

Fig. 10.5. In yab yum position a pillow under woman's buttocks helps to bring the bodies to a similar level so that they align at the genitals and hearts, which encourages circulation of energy.

there is a greater correspondence of the inner magnets within the bodies. The hearts meet through the chest and the breasts, and below there can be an almost magnetic lock of the organs, which then enables energy to ascend, circulate between the bodies, and expand beyond them. Yab yum can be sustained over a long period of time using different approaches to the breath, as suggested earlier. For instance, you can experiment with man breathing out of the penis and in through the heart, and woman breathing out through the breasts and in through the vagina.

Movement Is Part of Slow Sex

Movement is a blessing, movement is life. There is certainly no rule that says during slow sex there is no movement. It's more a question of how we move, as well as why. The basic inquiry is one of whether movement is mechanical or conscious, or if it is appropriate in any given moment, rather than the move being something habitual or deemed to be an essential ingredient of sex. In some moments stillness is appropriate, in others a slow movement is fitting, and in others a shift of position is required. What you do depends on the communication between the penis and vagina. Maybe an adjustment of the legs can deepen the penetration, or a small movement of the pelvis can open up a range of new inner sensations.

Movement is discussed in chapter 2, where it is mentioned, among other things, that an interesting aspect to explore is the basic motivation behind any movement. Why are we doing the movement? Is the movement for stimulating and building up excitement with orgasm in mind? Or do we move because we're wanting to increase awareness or physical comfort, or attempting to enhance pleasure through the correspondence of the penis and vagina?

Movements during slow sex occur in direct response to the present; they arise out of what is needed in the moment and are guided by the light of awareness.

Because they are not goal oriented (not moving toward climax in the future), slow sex movements are of quite a different quality than the movements in conventional sex; they are relaxed and leisurely, the moves evolve in a gradual, sensual, organic way. There is a sense of allowing it to happen, giving way and unfolding, rather than controlling the event according to our usual sexual routine or ideas.

Lust versus Passion

The difference between lust and passion is a matter of definition and requires some clarification. Many people think that in giving up orgasm they are giving up their passion, but this is not the case. Basically you are giving up lust. If you look closely at lust when you are caught up in it, it always has a direction. And this invites tension, expectation, and pressures that swamp the simple present moment. The movements will be building toward climax as the goal of the union. A fixation on the end point causes a lack of connection to the present, the orientation is in the future, sometimes subtle and sometimes not so subtle.

Slow sex is not lustful in the usual sense we understand (or experience) hot climactic sex. At the same time, slow sex can sometimes be full-on in a way that is utterly dynamic and involves big movements. But each movement comes from an inner place of stillness and is independent of the movement before it and of the movement after it. Each movement is complete in itself. The moves are not being stepped up to arrive at orgasm as final destination, but as a way of celebrating the present. This type of sexual experience is true passion—pure presence. Passion has no goal and leads nowhere.

You can be fully passionate and be totally unmoving. Or be utterly still and feel inwardly wild at the same time. Passion and authentic wildness are extremely conscious states that reflect tremendous inner vitality and sensitivity.

Sensational heat through the excitement of friction (repetitive in and out movements of the penis in the vagina) short-fuses the system because excitement so easily leads to orgasm. Friction for an extended time has to be used with caution in the sense that once we find ourselves on the roller coaster of excitement it's difficult (if not impossible) to find the awareness or wish to jump off the ride. That's why from the outset it's advisable to stay in the cooler zones of sexual connection where there is less excitement and stimulation, so you do not get hooked up with the need to climax. The coolness creates the sustainability. In addition, in the long term, mechanical friction between the genitals does, little by little, reduce their sensitivity. When sensitivity is lost, more sensation is required and then sensitivity suffers a further loss. To regain sensitivity also means to reside in the genitals in a cooler, calmer, more conscious way.

Instead of mechanical in-and-out movements there are an infinite number of subtle sideways or circular pelvic movements (especially of man) that will help the penis reach and probe into the deeper reaches of the vagina and touch all the surfaces, with very pleasurable effects. Woman can position her pelvis at interesting angles and then hold still so as to invite deeper exploration of the vaginal canal.

Recognizing the Urge for Orgasm

We all know intimately the urge for orgasm, but it is useful to be aware of it in the very moment the desire arises, when suddenly we become tense and switch into fast forward. It is not physically healthy to deliberately repress ejaculation or to repeatedly build tension up, then repress it again. So should ejaculation need to happen, let it be so. Basically orgasm is not wrong. What we are questioning is the conditioning that sex equals orgasm, and the habit of actively striving toward a climax. We are inadvertently creating tension and future goals when, in fact, we need to relax and be here to have elevated experiences.

There is an extremely creative option that you may want to try when faced with the desire for orgasm. When your desire arises, confront it with the totality of your awareness, the totality of your being. At the same time, relax the body utterly and completely. Breathe deeply into the belly and just be, alert in body and senses, present to the moment.

If you completely pull back from desire in the very instant it shows itself, a miraculous thing can happen. The energy that was moving outward is powerfully inverted and will implode within you, soon to rise up again through your core in a wave of vitality that becomes a tremendously empowering personal force.

You ascend to a higher octave, a rarer vibration beyond thought, where the bodies become spontaneous flowing forms and configurations.

If there is a decision for orgasm, don't go into it mechanically and blindly, but consciously and slowly, relaxing tensions, breathing deeply, using your inner eye of awareness to remain present to the unfolding. That very awareness of following the process and relaxing into it, rather than getting tense about it, will fundamentally transform the conventional orgasm experience.

Physical Comfort
Helps Relaxation and Sensitivity

Sustaining your practice also means you need to be able to sustain lying down in bed for longer periods, so be sure to take care of your physical needs. If there is discomfort in the legs, knees, hips, or back, it is time to change position. Otherwise the discomfort becomes a distraction and prevents you from settling into your body and your inner sensations.

Have on hand a selection of pillows of different shapes, sizes, and densities, which can be used to aid and support the postures, as illustrated in figures 10.6 and 10.7. (Also see figures 10.1 and 10.5 on pages 121 and 134 respectively.)

SITUATIONS AND ISSUES
THAT MAY ARISE DURING PRACTICE

It's helpful to know of common hindrances and difficulties that a couple can run into when practicing slow sex. Maybe you got off to a good start and things were going well for a period of time, but then one of you is feeling less satisfied with the practice. Or you are having difficulty keeping a commitment to the practice, you're meeting less often and finding excuses to cancel. Sometimes unexpected emotions arise and get in the way or your expectations are a little bit high, which blocks your awareness of the present moment. Below are some situations that you may find yourselves in, with guidelines on how to deal with them.

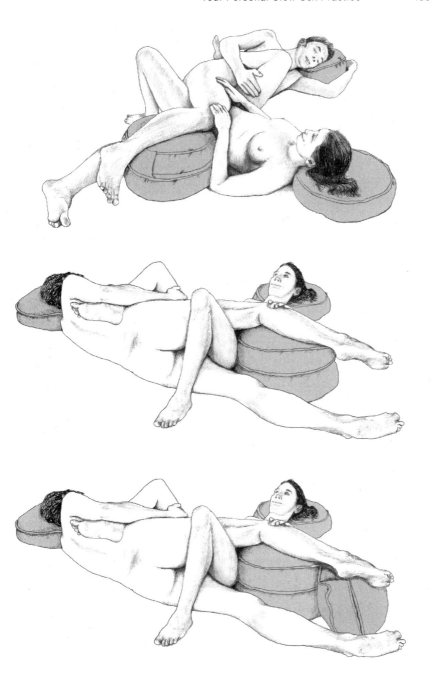

Fig. 10.6. In side-scissors position man can support his knee
and calf on a pillow. If desired, he can add another pillow
under his ankle and foot, as shown in the third image. As noted before,
both partners will be more comfortable with head support.

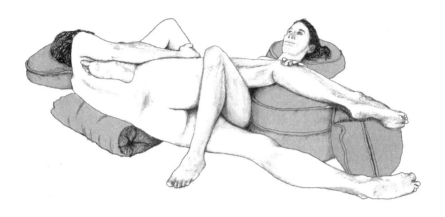

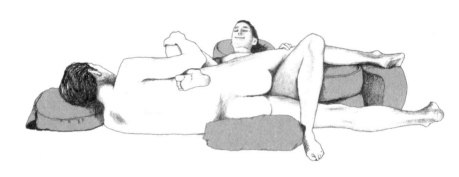

Fig. 10.7. To prevent himself from rolling backward in
side-scissors position, man can wedge a pillow support under
his back and pelvis. This is particularly helpful for sustained
soft penetration. The upper image shows support under both
back and hip; the lower image, hip support only.

No Sensitivity or Nothing Really Happens

Many people find that they don't have much sensitivity in the beginning, and the best approach is to accept the situation as it is. Look, it is going to feel different without the usual excitement or stimulation, so take that into account and don't expect to feel the same thing or even anything like it. Don't give in to frustration because you are not getting what you usually get. It's different, and that is all. It takes patience and curiosity to discover the delights of the subtle inner world. Accepting the reality that you don't feel very much will help you to relax, because all acceptance leads to inner relaxation. When we are fighting against something, resisting it, denying it, we create tension that stops us from feeling. If you allow tears of sadness to flow you will notice how your sensitivity improves.

Something always happens, even if it is nothing. Becoming aware of this nothingness is already something.

Nothingness is not easy to accept because there is a deep fear of emptiness and not feeling anything. Fear is often the motivation for movement in sex, to build up feeling in the way of sensation. So when you go slow, and sometimes stop, it will be normal that you cannot easily feel into your genital tissues. In the past you have perhaps been more *around* your genitals, not really in them. In a way it can be difficult to believe that we are not fully sensitive in that part of the body, partly because we are pretty sensitive there for the purposes of conventional sex, and partly because it is difficult to believe that *you* might be insensitive.

In our retreats we always make a great effort to gently warn couples that they may not feel anything at first. We say so again and again during our talks so as not to create expectations and possible disappointment. Even so, after a few days individuals do come up to me looking really shaky and concerned, and share that they can't feel anything in their genitals. So even though we warn people, it is still difficult to accept (and take in) when lack of feeling happens to you.

Patience is needed. Not patience as a duty, tapping your fingers in the meantime, but patience as compassion, understanding, respect; honoring yourself, your body, your partner, your partner's body. With patience comes stillness and silence, relaxation into what is present in any given moment.

Confusion, Insecurity, Not Knowing

It's quite usual, as you start to change your style of sex, to feel that you don't know who you really are. You may feel confused and somewhat lost. When you are on a learning curve a bit of confusion helps, because it loosens up the ego, the personality structure, and you become more vulnerable. You can't expect to be fluent in something that has not been your experience, so a period of disorientation is a valid response to the situation. If you think back to when you first had sex, you probably felt insecure then as well. But now that terrain is traveled and you know your way around. Now you are learning a whole new way of having sex, and also having to unlearn many things you've learned accidentally, so it would almost be surprising if you didn't feel somewhat baffled.

Share your feelings of confusion and insecurity with your partner as soon as they come up. Don't postpone talking about them, otherwise you'll just feel more and more shaky. Once you express what you feel, having said it out loud will quickly make you feel more at ease and at home within yourself. With more slow sex practice and experience you will soon find yourself feeling more confident, clear, and secure.

One Person Feels Something
and the Other Does Not

It easily happens that one partner can feel more than the other—usually the woman—and this is quite understandable. Woman as the receptive force, the environment that man moves into, is bound to feel what enters her environment. Conversely, man needs time and practice to orient himself in the new environment. Where woman feels something taking place within her body she can communicate that to man (or vice versa if the situation is reversed and man feels more than woman). She can briefly share what she feels with the presence of the penis inside her. Her feedback can be tremendously reassuring for a man—it tells him that at least his woman can feel him, a fact not to be underestimated.

One Partner Is Better at Communicating

It is often the case that one of the two finds it easier to share and express what is felt, where, and when. Their gift of sharing will support and encourage the other partner to express themselves in words. Do not make differences such as these into problems; rather see how you can help and support each other. The communication also acknowledges your inner body, so you are informing not only your partner, but more importantly, your higher self. Learning to talk about your inner sensitivity is an art that can be learned.

One tip is to start with what is. Often people are more focused on what they think should be, and begin to perceive a lack of something instead of directing the attention to what is present in the moment. Share about simple things you observe in the body. The feelings don't have to be momentous or extraordinary, just what is there. When you acknowledge what is present, you nurture roots of pleasure in the body, and your sensitivity will grow as these roots slowly spread through you.

You Don't Feel Like Having Sex

Bodies always love to make conscious love; the mind is less willing. Often, as in many other situations, there is a natural resistance to stepping out of the mind and into the here and now. It's the mind that will find all kinds of excuses. In this situation you need to acknowledge that you are in resistance, deliberately step over your mind, and connect with each other. Pretty soon you will find that your body is extremely happy to be in that situation. And if it really does not feel as if genital union is appropriate, then you can continue to enjoy an hour or two of intimacy—touching, breathing, receptive vision, being present to your body and each other.

It may appear on the surface that the resistance is a resistance to sex. But in reality the resistance is to being in the present.

I discovered this through the practice of massage, which has been a passion of mine for more than thirty years. In spite of how much I enjoyed it, shortly before an appointment I would often begin to hope that the telephone would ring and my client announce a sudden cancellation. Of course this did not usually happen, and soon enough there would be a knock at the door and I would simply have to accept the situation and proceed accordingly. As soon as the person was on the table and I started oiling their body, I would naturally bring myself into the present by connecting with the skin, flow of my hands, and movements of my body. Within five minutes I would be in heaven, slipping and sliding my way through ninety minutes with ease and timeless joy.

Some years later I was very surprised to notice the same type of resistance coming up with my sex appointments. And again the same realization—resistance to being present, not to sex. And again the same experience. If I accepted the situation and connected with my body in the present, everything flowed easily and the experience was a pleasure. So the guideline is to avoid listening to your mind, which is capable of a thousand and one excuses, and use your body as a bridge to the mystery of the present.

If you are genuinely ill it is wise to respect the state of your body and give it time to heal. If there is a fever or anything really debilitating, sex is probably not advisable. However, there may be some states in which you do feel weak and tired and yet capable of slow sex, especially as no great energy output is required. You will be surprised to discover that afterward you are likely to feel much better, with more energy and an increased sense of well-being.

It's a very good idea to keep your planned dates. It may be that your partner is really counting on that date, and if you make excuses or don't show up, the other person may be disappointed and feel let down. Causing this type of disturbance is really not worthwhile or supportive, as it can take time to get back into equilibrium.

You (or Your Partner) Are Falling Asleep

If you are in a relaxed position, such as the scissors position used for soft penetration, it's easy to feel sleepy or actually even fall asleep. This is especially true for man because lying on the side reminds him of sleep. Whereas woman lies on her back where it is less easy to sleep. It's fine to allow yourself the space to rest deeply for a short time; a short sleep can be regenerating. Some couples remain connected throughout the night, and this is also fine if you are able to sustain the position and sleep at the same time. It's something I have never managed.

In general, though, during sex it's time to be awake and not asleep. You have designated a place and a time and you have a commitment. If you arrive at your appointment exhausted from the other commitments of your day, tired and in need of some sleep, it is better to rest for twenty minutes or so before you begin. Your partner can rest with you. Set an alarm clock, bearing in mind that a twenty-minute nap is usually more refreshing than a two-hour sleep.

It's helpful to know that the urge to sleep can be due not only to tiredness, but also to avoidance.

Overwhelming heaviness in the eyelids can sometimes be induced by reluctance to acknowledge deeper feelings that are coming to the surface, such as old unexpressed pain. The pull toward sleep is a defense mechanism to switch you off and keep you comfortable and undisturbed. When you notice something like this happening to you, the way through is to take a step deeper into yourself, delve into the buried feelings, and give way to them. Afterward you will feel much more present, alive, and loving. Prolific yawning is often another symptom of underlying feelings rising to the surface. The yawning reflex keeps feelings at bay.

One Wants to Move and the Other Doesn't

Sometimes during slow sex one person wants to be more still and the other wants a bit more action. It's generally more common that the woman is seeking stillness and the man wants movement, and this is probably because the female organ is a receptive organ and the male organ is a dynamic organ. However, the man has to discover how to be present and vital within the vagina as a dynamic, complementary force, rather than being dynamic in the way of literal activity, moving in and out. So there is a need for man to challenge himself a little in order to discover the true qualities of his penis. He also needs to develop compassion for woman and a greater understanding of her situation. Too often she has entered sex without her body being fully open, and she has pushed herself to please man to keep love in her life. Now finally, with a new understanding in hand, she is able to relax and receive—her true nature. Usually she will intuitively know this is the right way for her.

At the same time, and equally important, woman needs to understand that man is stepping down from a big performance program (as demanded by conventional sex), and have compassion for him. Also, he has been accustomed to a rubbing movement in order to feel his penis. Basically, when a movement is a conscious movement, it slows down and the whole quality changes including sensitivity. So you can agree on conscious movement, which is fair enough. After all, it's been the unconscious way that has usually made woman less available for sex in the past.

What a woman has to watch out for is her mind falling into resistance, repeating again and again to herself, "I don't like it." This attitude makes you internally tight and unreceptive, so for sure you will not like it! You have to dive into yourself and see what you can do to change the situation, rather than ask the other person to change, as in "Please slow down" or "Please stop." Too many instructions can make a person feel manipulated and controlled, which can lead to feeling wrong or unworthy.

**I discovered that if I put all my awareness into relaxation,
widening and receiving, especially in the vagina (instead of**

being caught up in the mind), the man would slow down enormously and even sometimes come to a wide-eyed standstill.

In this way woman does have a certain power as the receptive environment. A penis entering the space is immediately affected by the absorbent forces enveloping it, and it's better for her to direct her energies in this direction, see how she can directly transform the situation through awareness, rather than try to change her man.

You Feel Frustrated

Frustration can arise because things are different and you don't get what you are accustomed to getting from sex. Frustration can also happen because you expect too much or don't feel much. If so, definitely begin to do something with your own body every day, some kind of exercise that you enjoy. Become more alive to yourself. To increase sensitivity and awareness in your genitals you can also do a self-massage of your pelvic floor.

⊙ Exercise: Pelvic Floor Self-Massage

1. Lying on your back, knees up, hands between your legs, make small circular movements with your fingertips circling deep above, on, and below the pubic bone, spreading sideways to the sitz bones. Then turn onto your side and reach behind to massage the coccyx area.
2. Then, lying on your back again, give a deep massage to the muscles around your genitals. Take about an hour to work on the area, and repeat the massage several times over the next few weeks.

A self-massage done with gentle, loving hands will help to release tension and increase circulation and sensitivity in the pelvic region.

It's important to find some kind of balance in the engagement between the two of you—you don't want to get so frustrated that you get turned off, so you need to keep it interesting. And at the same time, become aware of how strong the sexual conditioning is, how strong the urge to do something in sex is, and how difficult it is to just be floating in it. You need to be willing to challenge your patterns in order to access your higher sexual potential. It takes time and practice to learn the knack, so keep it interesting for yourselves and be patient, loving, generous, and supportive.

Loss of Erection

Loss of erection is natural when stimulation is reduced, so it is helpful to accept active and passive phases of the penis, and to accept soft entry as a viable alternative. Man carries a lot of insecurity and fear around the whole erection issue because it's fragile. Usually when a man begins to lose his erection he feels very awkward about it, even embarrassed, and the last thing he really wants is for his woman to realize it. So a man often tries to cover up a diminishing erection by exciting or stimulating himself or woman in some way. A relaxed penis is an equally valid instrument and it continues to have dynamic properties, however many men consider the erect version of the penis as being *the* penis. They believe a flaccid penis is of no real consequence, where soft sadly equals impotence.

Instead of feeling shame and fear around loss of erection (and trying to get it back), it is far better for a man to allow his penis to relax and stay within the vagina (or use soft entry), and at the same time connect with (be aware of and true to) his real feelings, which may be insecurity, weakness, or a feeling of helplessness.

Feeling these feelings can be a kind of small death. There may be sadness and tears, or not knowing, accompanied by shaking and shivering. Expressing the deeper fears that underly loss of erection is a form of healing, cleansing, and empowerment that establishes a man more deeply in his authentic male authority.

Expecting Results

People often ask, "How long before we can expect ecstasy?" Such expectations show that you are standing in your own way. Ecstasy can never be a demand or an expectation; it's a blessing and a gift. You have to create the situation and be an invitation for bliss to descend upon you. It needs receptivity and preparation. There are some prerequisites to meeting the Divine—naturalness, egolessness, and timelessness. Ecstasy happens when immersed in the present, not absent through being expectant. And in any event, many thrilling moments of delight and pleasure are possible every time you get together.

People often think that ecstasy is something hot and overwhelming, but this is not really true. Ecstasy is, in fact, exceptionally cool and peaceful, and arises when there is a silent receptivity, porousness, and ease.

We cannot expect bliss from the first footstep we take on the journey. Many steps have to be taken, but these are not arduous; the way is one of fun, curiosity, and exploration. Become sensitive and attuned to yourself on the cellular level first. Put the foundations in place and build on that solid base.

Making Rules Out of Tools

A very common error is to turn tools into rules. When we get serious, tools become rules and exploration is no longer possible. Women, especially, tend to point their fingers—do this, don't do this. Loving, playful cooperation is absolutely essential, otherwise we don't get anywhere.

Trial and error is what you are after. Teach yourself, explore, and establish the truth of each tool instead of making it a rule. Finding the truth also means exploring tried and tested ways (as in conventional sex), so do not deny your past experience. Use the past as a bridge to the present. Return to known experiences in order to discover the truth, and don't rush to conclusions, as in, "It's like this because of that." Check it out again and again, and see if the same holds true over time. Only then is a truth truly your truth—when it has stood the test of time.

Lack of Time

The time factor is a common complaint from couples. Even with the best of intentions, between the joys and stresses of family life and work life there is rarely enough space for slow sex dates. In the end you simply have to carve time for yourselves as a couple and at least find time for the slow sex quickie now and then. Love has to be given some priority. Consciously creating love through slow sex will support you personally and as a couple, and put you in a better position to handle every other aspect of your life.

Arguing, Discussing, or Fighting

If you find yourself in some kind of argument, discussion, or blaming mode while supposedly having sex, then it's best to take some space apart from each other. Or it may be more subtle—you may notice some kind of negative or unloving charge (hidden or not) in your communication. If there's any kind of emotion in the air, then sex can easily move in the direction of excitement and discharge as a way of eliminating the emotional tension. Best is to tell your partner what's happening with you, using simple, first-person words such as, "I feel emotional," or "I feel disconnected from myself and you." Then separate physically (after agreeing that you will meet again later), find a place to be alone, and do something active with your body.

Do something physically strenuous, and with intention, to rid yourself of the accumulated tension. When you have come back to yourself and can feel your heart again, return to your partner. Usually there will be an immediate sense of connection, but if for any reason you continue to feel slightly separate, you may need to move a bit more. Whatever you choose to do, do it with intention and self-awareness, not in a halfhearted way.

The danger of staying in the same place, not separating, is that the talking and arguing will be prolonged, perhaps going around in circles for hours. The unhappiness and tension that has arisen (for whatever reason) has to be dealt with differently in order to protect and preserve your love. If you continue fighting, too easily things escalate and hurtful, revengeful things are said to each other, which is a much less effective way to rid the system of tension. So if you hear yourself using phrases like "you always" or "you never," this is a signal that you have moved from connection into disconnection. Or if you notice you can't look your partner in the eyes, this too is a sign that the connection is out of order. (For more on this subject see below, "Separating Love from Emotion," and the book *Tantric Love: Feeling versus Emotion— Golden Rules to Make Love Easy* by Diana and Michael Richardson.) Recognize what's happening, announce it, and separate briefly to get a handle on the situation without acting it out on your partner. And then afterward come back together again.

DEEPENING YOUR SLOW SEX PRACTICE

Your experience will deepen through regular and frequent practice, not just leaving it for now and then (although now and then is infinitely better than not at all). You may reach various plateaus, which is perfectly fine, and also rewarding and beneficial. Regular meetings give rise to a refining of the polarity within and between your bodies— male more male, female more female. You become more finely tuned as time passes.

Unlike conventional sex where the thrills tend to dry up over time, slow sex is sustainable over many, many years and encourages togetherness. Sex can be a cohesive force.

This bonding element alone speaks loud and clear for the value of slow sex. I hear from so many couples after our retreats that the only reason they are still together is because they began practicing slow sex. Through the awareness required they came back into connection with themselves, and through that, with each other. The awareness made it possible and easy to be able to continue a loving relationship in happiness and harmony. When the level of awareness between any two people is raised, then love is the alchemical by-product.

PENETRATING INNOCENCE

Stay light, easy, and playful. These qualites of innocence will support you. A sense of humor is tantamount to a best friend when you explore sex. Very amusing situations can arise so the capacity to be light and see the funny side of things helps. A sense of humor gives you perspective on the situation; you are less identified with what is taking place. A sense of humor definitely means being able to laugh at yourself. When we are lacking in humor it may be because we are somehow trapped in the mind and identified with our sexual selves, our performance, or how the other person perceives us as a lover. Avoid taking yourself too seriously and don't get serious about what you are doing. Make it a play, a dance. Be easygoing with yourself and your partner. Life and love are an unfolding mystery and adventure, so it doesn't help to get too serious about them.

What is essential is sincerity of the heart, not seriousness of the mind. Sincerity keeps to the commitment, gives rise to curiosity and willingness, and knows the value of love.

Entering the inner dimensions and realms of the body is basically a feminine search. The spiritual inquiry is a feminine one because it looks inward; both man and woman are engaging with the feminine. This is an essential balance to our very extroverted, masculine, outward-oriented society with its material, external values. As a general shift, humanity needs to turn back inward to access resources that lie within and have sustainable value beyond the material.

When the dynamic and receptive sexual forces resting deep within are allowed to express themselves in slow sex, tremendous healing and regeneration is possible, both individually and collectively. Engaging in slow sex enables your system to come into natural flow and balance. As you heal and harmonize yourselves you will generate a powerful positive energy that becomes a contribution to society at large.

Developing Presence

Our first effort must be to arrive in the present. The present moment is most easily found in your body. Through being aware in the body, the senses, the breath, and the inner world, you being to develop the quality of presence. This quality has the capacity to develop and grow to the extent that your presence begins to have an impact on others and alchemically draw them into the here and now.

> **Don't be concerned as to whether your partner is present or not; rather, look to see if *you* are present or not. And find ways to intensify your presence (using your awareness) so that it energetically draws and engages your partner.**

I found it a great help to always try to change myself first, before considering what I could ask my partner to change. It's not that you deny your needs or your truth, but first and foremost you turn back toward yourself and become curious as to what you can influence through your awareness and relaxation. For me, doing so has always had magical results.

A Shift from Doing to Being

The body is the bridge to the being, and when you relax into your being, you naturally connect with the source of love within yourself. The source of love is within you, not outside you. At times you may decide to drop verbal communication or close your eyes, because you have reached a stage where you can hold the awareness in the present and for a change wish to enjoy silence, closed eyes, and just being.

There are quite a few inner doings that can go on while you

are being in your body. You might want to experiment with some of the following:

- Bring your awareness to your perineum (man) or breasts (woman) and notice what takes place on a subtle energy level.
- Travel internally with your breath and assist it in reaching deep into the genital tissues.
- Breathe incredibly softly with your awareness at the nasal openings and see how you can enter into your breath.
- Curl the tip of your tongue upward until it touches the roof of your mouth, and feel what inner connection happens when you leave it there.
- Bring your awareness to the third eye (midline forehead, just above the eyebrows) and feel the inner expansion.
- Hold the awareness in the solar plexus and see how a certain spontaneity arises in your body, or in the connection between you and your partner.

Little tricks like these, connecting energy circuits or connecting to energy points (using the awareness), will often intensify inner sensations and sensitivities, and they are great to play around with and explore. At the same time, getting too involved with this inner point or that inner point can turn into a subtle form of doing and create a slight but significant level of absence. So this by-product has to be balanced by simply being present to what *is* in the body.

Spontaneous Erection and Orgasmic Experiences

Spontaneous erection, one where the penis spirals upward by itself inside the vagina, can happen at any time. This phenomenon is based on a magnetic type of interaction between the penis and vagina's dynamic and receptive forces, as we discussed in more detail in chapter 4. Avoid having expectations. It may happen, it may not happen. Maybe today, maybe tomorrow. But do not use spontaneous erection as any kind of measure of success. Do not expect anything to happen because expectations form subtle barriers that block your potential experience. Expectation involves thought and judgment and removes you from your inner connection to the body. Spontaneous erection will usually be a by-product of deep merging with body and senses; it can never be a goal because it is an outcome of a certain constellation of factors. You can only create the situation and settle ever more deeply into your body.

Orgasmic states can arise for both man and woman, but they cannot in any way be engineered or expected. In the orgasmic state you experience an expansion beyond the physical boundaries where you come to exist as pure boundless energy through a deep relaxation and inner merging.

SEPARATING LOVE FROM EMOTION

Love is not an emotion, it is a state of being. Love is tremendous insight, clarity, sensitivity, and awareness, and these intrinsic qualities grow when we relax back into the body to touch the source of love that resides in the being. Taking responsibility for negative emotions and emotionality is a big step in maturity that permits us to behave as adults and not five-year-olds. With taking responsibility comes a newfound freedom in which we are able to preserve love and leave behind unhelpful patterns. A slow sex practice will definitely bring more harmony and reduce the level of emotionality between partners.

Expressing Feelings and Sharing Your Needs

It becoms necessary to communicate your needs and not expect your partner to intuit them. Sometimes it is difficult to admit to our needs, let alone express them, but if you don't tell your partner what does or doesn't suit you, you risk feeling unhappy a bit later on—like a backlash. Not getting needs fulfilled is a big source of our unhappiness and emotions. By speaking up in sex it is possible to eliminate at least one source of ongoing unhappiness and discontent.

When feelings rise to the surface, give way to them, let them move through you. Or tell your partner what you are feeling, making sure to talk only about yourself and avoid any form of subtle blaming or making your partner responsible for what you feel. Releasing or sharing old unexpressed aspects of yourself is integrating and deeply healing. Through purifying the tensions of old feelings that are stored in your body, you transform like a caterpillar becoming a butterfly.

The Difference between Feelings and Emotions

If you don't express your feelings or share your needs it is highly likely that sooner or later you will get emotional. Feelings and emotions are not the same and knowing the difference is life changing.

A feeling arises for expression out of the present moment, but when it remains unexpressed, the energy can turn in to negative emotion.

That means that feelings we do *not* express in the present get stored inside us, accumulate with time, and cause disturbances. You will know the moment you are emotional because there are certain distinct signs or symptoms that help you to recognize what is going on.

For the brief period of time when we are emotional, we are unconsciously caught up in the past, and not really anchored in the present and in reality. You begin to experience distance or a sense of separation from your partner (and also from yourself), whereas earlier you were feeling connected. When everything was rosy in the present there was the experience of connection—you were with the perfect person. Now, however, you may suddenly find yourself feeling far away and finding fault with your partner in some way, blaming them for this or that.

These swings in mood happen because from time to time our stored, unexpressed feelings get triggered, in and out of sex. And what leads us into trouble is that we have a *multitude* of unexpressed feelings, given that we live in a society where expressing genuine heartfelt feelings is not really okay. So most of us (and especially men) repress many of our feelings. As a result of centuries of repression, human beings have the tendency to be pretty emotional. All the unexpressed feelings remain in the system and go slightly sour, and when provoked in any way (even the slightest nudge can start a fist fight) they pop up and express themselves. The difficulty lies in the fact that the old unexpressed feelings have become toxins in the system, which explains why so often a person becomes so destructive or so vengeful when caught in the emotional state.

People sometimes do and say dreadful things to each other when they are experiencing a wave of emotion. And the toxic vengeful quality of emotion is the reason why whenever you recognize that you are emotional, you must literally tell your partner, "I am emotional." And then, to avoid further possibly hurtful words, leave the room.

Instead of venting your emotion on your partner, do something physical to burn up the emotion that has become active in your system. This really simple solution may appear *too* simple, but it invariably works. Afterward, when you return to your partner, the wall that was separating you has probably come down. If not, that's your signal to go and do some more work on yourself. Taking responsibility in this way means that you save yourselves the pain of going through many emotional upheavals that are destructive to your love connection. After too many fights the repairs start to take more time and be more temporary. Love slowly begins to erode and slip out of our hands. The toxins produced by too many fights, or one fight too many, has been the cause of many a couple finally separating.

Love is precious and we have to protect it from the destructive effects of overwhelming and inconstant emotion. Knowing how to tell the difference between the two very different states of emotion and feeling can save your relationship.

Deepening Polarity and Healing of the Penis and Vagina

As a couple opens to slow sex, the genitals go through a purifying, refining, and balancing process. Pain in the male or female genitals is sometimes indicative of old tensions leaving the body, yet another expression of buried and unresolved feelings. Be aware that healing or detoxification happens at any time and in many forms. For instance, nausea or vomiting, loose stools, headaches or migraines, toothache, exhaustion, boils or pimples, irregular heartbeat, or feeling very weak.

It's common for some women to experience pain in the vagina during sex and, regrettably, they accept it as part of the package. Some women will even fake pleasure by making suitable sounds when in reality sex feels painful to them. As a woman gets older and enters menopause, she frequently will report pain upon penetration or dryness of the tissues, so much that she can no longer have sex. Slow sex, however, is possible and enjoyable.

Sometimes during sex a woman will become aware of hidden pains or numb places at the entrance, along the sides, or deep in the higher part of the vagina.

Pain and deadness usually represent old wounds or memories stored in the tissue. Pain is positive in the sense that it acts as a door to the past and the tension accumulated there.

The powerful and healing effects of conscious sustained penetration are described in detail in chapter 8.

Opening to and giving way to buried feelings can be an effective way to release physical pain in the body, especially pain in the genital region. If you have a pain that suddenly arises and persists, especially after sex, always look to see if there is an emotional component hiding behind it. Perhaps there is some sadness, anger, or anxiety that you are holding under the surface. Allowing old feelings heals, balances, and sensitizes.

Men can also experience uncomfortable pain when they start to have slow, conscious sex. Pain in the groin, testicles, or penis is usually an indication of previously held tension being released and purified from the system. (Please note that ejaculation control by repression is not recommended, as mentioned earlier. Repressing ejaculation will also lead to pain and tension, but this is due to congestion and not because of purification.)

Sustained penetration can become a style of sex, with or without erection. The opposite poles spend simple time together and gradually become more attuned and alive.

RAISING CONSCIOUSNESS

In many ways, mastering slow sex is really a matter of unlearning a certain behavior and learning another one. You are installing consciousness in a place where expression has been more automatic, mechanical, and unconscious. So transforming unconsciousness into consciousness is a great shift and gift for your life, a blessing intended for you by the Creator.

Afterward Is Your Teacher

Essentially you have to teach yourself the conscious way. Learning is not going to happen just by reading and thinking about it; rediscovery can only happen through practice—hands-on experience. What you learn from yourselves is revealed by how you feel after you have had sex. Afterward is your teacher and shows you the way.

Intentionally begin to observe yourself after you have finished making love. How do you feel? Pay attention to immediately after, a short time later, and even a couple of days later. The tendency is to evaluate the high point—the climax—but we do not really observe ourselves during the minutes and hours beyond the moment of orgasm. Watching yourself afterward helps you to put together a new picture of sex. If you notice after slow sex, even while you may have "missed" some aspects of the fast approach (such as orgasm), that you feel more at ease in yourself, more loving, more nourished, then this feedback is teaching you something about the nature of exchange. If you perhaps observe that you feel brittle, abandoned, or lonely, it's good to look back at that as well. What did you do and how did you do it? Do you notice a connection between what you do and how you feel afterward?

> My partner and I tell people in our groups that "afterward" is their teacher, we are not. Both of us have certainly found that observation of the period of time after sex, even days later, has been the greatest teacher thus far.

Teach yourself through asking, "How was it?" Teach yourself how as you go along, by trial and error. Starting happens by getting down to doing it, and in your own individual way. Approach it with a sense of adventure, interested in what lies on the horizon.

Becoming Messengers of Love

Slow sex is an inquiry; you begin to examine sex. Answers will come to you, like the slow dawning of the day; you don't have to know everything in advance. Wanting questions answered in full before being willing to step out is not realistic. You might hear something said, but to make it your own truth, the experience has to be lived, and the truth verified.

Sincerity and general sensitivity in the body, especially the genital union, can produce transforming higher states of consciousness.

> Ecstasy is not, however, the new goal that replaces the old goal of orgasm. It cannot be seen in this way because ecstasy only shows itself when there is a dropping of goals, a diving into the present, and a dissolving into the infinite inner cosmos.

Recall the three beautiful elements to the experience of blissfulness mentioned: egolessness, naturalness, and timelessness. Egolessness means there is no "I." Naturalness means you surrender to the intelligence of your body. Timelessness means you slip into the present, and therefore completely out of time. Bliss can also happen without a partner, such as when alone enraptured by nature, and many people have had such an experience. So we cannot do bliss, we can only humbly and reverently create the situation that allows bliss. Sex definitely offers the perfect situation for exploring these elements, and it is perhaps one of the easiest, because the central theme reduces itself down to how you do something, and not what you do. Attributes such as innocence, sincerity, compassion, and courage are the qualities to pursue in order to elevate consciousness.

You don't need advanced techniques. The ever-deepening experience of penetrating your inner world can accompany you for the rest of your life. It's an experience that evolves with time and practice. Sex gets more simple, sensitivity grows, and you transform as time goes on. Slow sex becomes a practice involving a finely tuned awareness with positive, uplifting, long-term benefits that generally increase the quality of love and of life. While slow sex encourages togetherness, it also encourages aloneness and independence. You begin to feel complete, whole, and integrated, happier in and with yourself.

As you grow together you also grow as individuals, and your male and female poles come into balance. And the curious thing about the inner balancing of masculine and feminine energies within yourself is that you don't need to do anything with the opposite pole. You need only live and explore your male qualities as man, or your female qualities as woman. Living these aspects will alchemically establish the equal and opposite pole within you. Man by being more male accesses his feminine qualities, while woman through being more female accesses her masculine qualities.

Your inner flow of magnetism comes to life in such a way that energy can stream within you as a form of inner sex. This means you can circulate energy within yourself and continue the inner process of transformation that you have started together. The capacity to circulate vitality within yourself is the most evolved form of sex given to human beings, so it is something that can be done alone or in each other's company. You may already feel some streaming within; if not, visualization works very well, as it helps to awaken the energy.

Through practicing slow sex you will come to see and understand that sex is not what it seems to be on the surface. Any inherited preconceptions and ideas of sex are mostly false, and these misunderstandings form a screen between you and the real power of sex.

Through sexual exploration you will discover that the true function of slow sex is to bring more love into being. In this way each and every person can be a messenger of love by creating love and offering it to the world. Likewise, a couple can become a positive force in the community as generators of love and light.

Man's deepest wish is to be loved by woman, just as woman's deepest wish is to be loved by man. When you discover the how of love, then love is easily sustained. Couples begin to value, support, and appreciate each other as equal yet fundamentally opposite and complementary forces.

If there is any hope for humanity, perhaps the only genuine hope is that man and woman find peace with each other. Practicing sex in a conscious, slow way builds bridges of communication that kindle the flame of peace, enabling them to live as a cohesive force enjoying physically and spiritually uplifting lives.

The end of the story is that there has to be a drastic turnaround in the way people use their sexual energy. A few innocent, simple sexual steps are all it takes to initiate a journey back home to oneself, in accord with nature and the cosmic plan. There has to be a ripening and maturing process, whereby sex incorporates the universal metabolic enhancers so that the higher dimensions can easily be accessed and revealed. Slow sex is simple, sustainable, and life affirming, and enables us to be radiant purveyors of light, love, and peace on Earth.

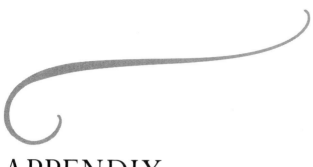

APPENDIX
True Male and Female Qualities versus Conditioned Distortions

Pages 164 and 165 present tables that list male and female qualities. The column on the left in each table lists the essential deep-seated qualities of man or woman. The column on the right lists the outcome or pattern when these intrinsic qualities become (unconsciously) distorted through sexual and societal conditioning. Because all human beings carry male and female poles within themselves, it can also happen that a man may sometimes demonstrate distorted female qualities, while at times a woman may display distorted male qualities. Approaching sex in a conscious, slow way leads to personal purification and healing of the body and psyche, promoting spontaneous inner balancing and integration.

TRUE MALE QUALITIES
VERSUS CONDITIONED DISTORTIONS

TRUE QUALITIES	CONDITIONED DISTORTIONS
Pure consciousness	Unconsciousness
Power	Abuse of power, domination
Presence	Absence
Strength	Hardness, violence
Clarity	Judgment
Assuredness	Aggression
Directed action, dynamic	Activity, restless, doing
Creativity	Achievement, ambition
Will	Stubbornness
Courage	Compensation, arrogance
Leadership	Control, politics, law and order
Protector	Patriarch
Authority	Authoritarian
Wildness	Brutality
Clear mind	Arrogance
Charisma	Sexual manipulation
Sun, seed of creation	Sunburn, ecological destruction
Expression, articulation	Pomposity, uncouth behavior
Heartfelt, compassionate	Selfish, egoistic
Differentiation	Separation

TRUE FEMALE QUALITIES
VERSUS CONDITIONED DISTORTIONS

TRUE QUALITIES	CONDITIONED DISTORTIONS
Unconditional love	Love with conditions
Pure energy	Hysterical
Electromagnetic field of attraction	Projects attractiveness
Appreciates inner beauty	Attached to outer appearance
Receptivity	Passivity
Loving	Jealous, manipulative, possessive
Softness	Weakness
Relaxed, nondoing	Inertia, laziness, collapse
Earth, manifesting creation, nurturing	Overbearing, interfering
Embracing	Overwhelming
Ability to surrender	Submissive, giving in, losing self
In contact with feelings	Emotional swings, sentimental, moody
Sensitive	Oversensitive, prickly, brittle
Nesting instinct	Obsessed with security
Intuitive, psychic	Suspicious, fearful
Enveloping	Sucking, taking
Sweetness	Hardness, stoniness
Silently strong	Masochistic, holding back energy
Connecting	Invasive
Trusting, allowing	Controlling, indecisive, lacking initiative
Connected to the universe	Spaced out, lacking personal boundaries

BOOKS
AND RESOURCES

David, Marc. *The Slow Down Diet: Eating for Pleasure, Energy, and Weight Loss*. Rochester, Vt.: Healing Arts Press, 2005.

Honoré, Carl. *In Praise of Slowness: Challenging the Cult of Speed*. New York: HarperCollins, 2005.

Lloyd, J. William. *The Karezza Method or Magnetation: The Art of Connubial Love*. Charleston, S.C.: Forgotten Books, 2008. (Originally printed privately for the author in 1931.)

Richardson, Diana. *The Heart of Tantric Sex: A Unique Guide to Love and Sexual Fulfilment*. Alresford, Hants, United Kingdom: "O" Books, 2002. (Originally published in 1999 as *The Love Keys: The Art of Ecstatic Sex*.)

———. *Tantric Love Letters: A Collection of Experiences, Questions, and Answers*. Alresford, Hants, United Kingdom: "O" Books, 2011.

———. *Tantric Orgasm for Women*. Rochester, Vt.: Destiny Books, 2004.

Richardson, Diana, and Michael Richardson. *Making Love: What You Should Always Have Known About Sex*. DVD of a live talk. Voice tracks in English and German. Cologne, Germany: Innenwelt Verlag, 2011. Available at www.livingloveshop.com.

———. *MaLua Light Meditation for Women*. Guided breast meditation CD with music, available in English and German. Cologne, Germany: Innenwelt Verlag, 2009.

———. *Tantric Love: Feeling versus Emotion—Golden Rules to Make Love Easy*. Alresford, Hants, United Kingdom: "O" Books, 2010. (Originally published in German in 2006.)

———. *Tantric Sex for Men: Making Love a Meditation*. Rochester, Vt.: Destiny Books, 2010.

———. *Time for Touch: Massage Using Awareness and Relaxation*. Instructional DVD. Voice tracks in English and German. Cologne, Germany: Innenwelt Verlag, 2010. Available at www.livingloveshop.com.

Robinson, Marnia. *Cupid's Poisoned Arrow: From Habit to Harmony in Sexual Relationships*. New York: Random House, 2009.

Rosenberg, Marshall. *Nonviolent Communication: A Language of Life*. Encinitas, Calif.: Puddle Dancer Press, 2003.

Stockham, Alice Bunker. *Karezza: Ethics of Marriage*. Charleston, S.C.: Forgotten Books, 2008. (Originally published in 1903.)

Versluis, Arthur. *The Secret History of Western Sexual Mysticism: Sacred Practices and Spiritual Marriage*. Rochester, Vt.: Destiny Books, 2008.

"MAKING LOVE"
A Tantra Meditation Retreat for Couples

The author and her partner, Michael, offer weeklong retreats in Switzerland that guide couples into the art of slow, conscious sex. For more information about their work please visit their websites listed below.

www.livinglove.com
www.love4couples.com

You may contact Diana and Michael by e-mail at the following address.

info@livinglove.com

BOOKS OF RELATED INTEREST

Tantric Sex for Men
Making Love a Meditation
by Diana Richardson and Michael Richardson

Tantric Orgasm for Women
by Diana Richardson

The Complete Illustrated Kama Sutra
Edited by Lance Dane

Healing Love through the Tao
Cultivating Female Sexual Energy
by Mantak Chia

Tao Tantric Arts for Women
Cultivating Sexual Energy, Love, and Spirit
by Minke de Vos
Foreword by Mantak Chia

Sacred Relationships
The Practice of Intimate Erotic Love
by Anaiya Sophia and Padma Aon Prakasha

Lingam Massage
Awakening Male Sexual Energy
by Michaela Riedl and Jürgen Becker

Yoni Massage
Awakening Female Sexual Energy
by Michaela Riedl

Inner Traditions • Bear & Company
P.O. Box 388
Rochester, VT 05767
1-800-246-8648
www.InnerTraditions.com

Or contact your local bookseller